MW01265441

The Beginner's Guide to Essential Oils & Aromatherapy

Written by Meghan Foster

This is Book 1 of the **Essentially Yours** series of books.

<u>Disclaimer:</u>

The information contained in this book is for general information purposes only.

While we endeavor to keep the information up to date and correct, we make no representations or warranties of any kind, express or implied, about the completeness, accuracy, reliability, suitability or availability with respect to the book or the information, products, services, or related graphics contained in the book for any purpose. Any reliance you place on such information is therefore strictly at your own risk.

None of the information in this this book is meant to be construed as medical advice. Always consult with a medical profession prior to making any dietary changes in your life.

None of the health benefits mentioned in this book pertaining to use of essential oils have been evaluated or approved by the FDA. Do not use essential oils in place of medical treatment, nor should they be used to treat, diagnose, cure or prevent any disease, ailment or injury. Use essential oils at your own risk.

Contents

What Are Essential Oils?

The scientific community defines *essential oils* as natural aromatic compounds that are contained within plants. In simple terms, essential oils are the compounds that give plants their characteristic scents. They're contained in all parts of the plant, including the roots, stems, seeds, flowers and wood. Some portions of the plant contain higher concentrations of essential oils than others, which is the reason why you smell a floral scent when you smell a flower, but don't get the same fragrance when you smell the stems or branches.

If you've ever stopped to smell the roses or wandered through a eucalyptus grove, you've smelled the aromatic fragrance of essential oils. Bend a lime peel back and forth and you'll see little geysers of liquid spray out. This liquid will smell strongly of lime and what you're witnessing is little geysers of essential oil erupting from the peel. The scent of a sprig of mint and the pungent aroma of fresh basil are other smells you're probably familiar with that can be attributed to essential oils. If you pick a leaf from a mint plant and rub it between your fingers, you'll release some of the essential oils from within the leaf and the smell of mint will get stronger.

Essential oils aren't there just to make a plant smell good. They play a number of key biological roles. Some oils are designed by nature to deter pests, while others are present to attract beneficial insects like pollinators and the predatory insects that prey on pests. Some oils may even play a key role in keeping plants healthy and fighting off disease. The antifungal and antibacterial nature of the oils gives plants a natural defense against harmful microorganisms that would otherwise do them harm. There are even some oils like eucalyptol and camphor that can be released by plants into the soil to prevent other plants from growing nearby.

The next time you smell a plant, consider that it isn't just the scent of the plant you're smelling. It's the aromatic essence, or the essential oils, of the plant that are making their way to your nose. In addition to playing key roles in the survival of plants, a number of essential oils are beneficial to humans when applied to the skin or inhaled. We've yet to unlock all of the benefits of essential oils, but there are many practical uses that are already known, some of which have been known for thousands of years and others we've just recently discovered.

What Is Aromatherapy?

Aromatherapy is defined as the use of essential oils to promote better health of the mind, body and soul. For those who practice aromatherapy, it's part art, part science and part tradition, as the use of plant oils is based in science, but dates back thousands of years. It's a means through which the individual can get in touch with their inner self and holistically rebalance their health and well-being through use of natural compounds. Aromatherapy is both a proactive and preventative approach to promoting better health of the mind, the body and the soul.

There are a number of ways essential oils act upon the body when they're used for aromatherapy, including the following:

- **Essential oils contain a number of compounds that are beneficial to the human body.**
- **They're absorbed into the skin and can act on the immediate area where they've been applied. They're also picked up by capillaries beneath the skin and are able to travel throughout the blood stream and can be used by the body as needed.**
- **When the oils are inhaled, the fragrance of the oils can be used to invoke a certain mental response.**
- **When the oils are inhaled, small particles of oil are absorbed into the blood stream and travel throughout the body.**

Essential oils are entirely natural and non-invasive. Those who use them don't seek to mask the symptoms of a health issue. Instead, they go straight to the source of the problem by boosting the body's natural ability to heal and maintain itself. You probably aren't going to be able to completely eliminate the need for modern medicine from your life, but there are a growing number of people who are realizing a variety of benefits stemming from use of essential oils.

Here are just some of the many things essential oils are known to do:

- Kill bacteria and prevent new bacteria from forming.
- Prevent fungal growth and aid with fungal infections.
- Reduce inflammation, both inside and outside the body.
- Prevent oxidation.
- Kill parasites.
- Prevent sepsis in wounds.
- Ease muscle spasms.
- Help prevent viruses.
- Boost the immune system.
- Soothe aches and pains.
- Stimulate the mind and body.
- Soothe frayed nerves.
- Break up congestion and help with respiratory problems.
- Improve circulation.
- Improve digestive health.

- Improve mental stability.
- Improve organ function.
- Protect damaged skin.
- Hair care.
- Pain relief.
- Relaxation.

While there's no single oil that'll allow you to reap all of these benefits at once, oil blends can be created that will allow you to stack a number of benefits on top of one another. Oil blends will be covered in detail in a future chapter.

We've Been Using Them a Long Time

Travel back through the annals of time and you'll uncover countless points in the history of man where plant oils have been put to use to improve the health of the people using them. While you won't see the term "essential oils" being used in older literature to describe the use of plant oils, what you will uncover are a variety of plant oils being used as far back as 7,000 B.C. That's right, even our ancient ancestors were aware of the powers of essential oils and weren't past blending them with animal fat and rubbing them into wounds.

The vast majority of cultures have put essential oils to use at one time or another. The ancient Egyptians used them extensively, as did the Chinese, Greeks, Romans and the Persians. They were used for everything from medicine to flavoring foods and were even put to use as health and beauty products. The Greeks ranked amongst the first people to use essential oils for their scents and they incorporated them into massages in order to reap many of the same benefits they're used for in modern times.

It didn't take long to discover plant oils could be extracted from the plants that contained them using methods such as pressing and distillation, which are still in use in some areas of the world today. This allowed for the collection of larger amounts of concentrated oils that could then be sold and traded on the open market. Essential oils became highly sought after commodities and many a ship was lost trying to navigate treacherous trade routes that would take them to a supplier of exotic oils like frankincense and myrrh. Some of the largest trade deals at the time were hammered out to ensure ample amounts of precious essential oils would be delivered in a constant supply. Much of the exploration of the world was commissioned by kings looking for easier trade routes and faster access to exotic spices and oils.

As trade routes were established and essential oils became more available, they rapidly spread across the globe. At first, the use of essential oils was limited to those in power and the rich who could afford them, but they soon became ingrained in everyday life. Massage oils were invented, oils were taken internally to help ease a number of health problems and religions began integrating them into their rituals. Essential oils are mentioned in a number of instances in the Bible, and most well-known of which are frankincense and myrrh, the two oils given to baby Jesus by the wise men when they arrived to celebrate his birth.

Excuse the pun, but essential oils played, well, an essential role in medicine for thousands, if not tens of thousands, of years, but fell out of favor as modern medicine moved to forefront. They were all but forgotten in the Western world until René-Maurice Gattefossé, a French chemist, burned his hand badly in the late 1930's and dipped into the only thing he had on hand—pure lavender oil. He was shocked at how quickly the lavender oil provided relief from the burns and healed his wounds with minimal scarring and went on to invent "Aromatherapie," which was the predecessor to modern aromatherapy. He published a number of books on the subject and became one of the leaders in the modern aromatherapy movement.

Fast-forward to today and essential oils and aromatherapy are seeing something of a revival as a large number of people are seeking to return to the ways of old by using natural remedies and treatments instead of the harsh chemicals associated with modern medicine. They're turning to holistic health and natural treatments in an attempt to rebalance their body with nature instead of further tilting the imbalance by adding more chemicals to treat problems caused by other chemicals.

They Sound Great, but Are They Safe?

For the vast majority of people, there are a large number of essential oils that can safely be used for therapeutic purposes. To be clear, there is a small percentage of the population that can't handle essential oils. Some can't tolerate certain oils, while others can't tolerate any type of essential oil at all. The reaction these people have when exposed to essential oils can range from mild to severe. It can be similar to the reaction experienced during food allergies, in that the body initiates an immune response when it comes in contact with the oils, which shouldn't come as a surprise since a number of the plants the oils come from are used for food.

Localized rashes, swelling, itching and a number of other symptoms can occur. When the reaction is minor, you might be able to wait a day or two and the symptoms will go away. If the reaction is severe, immediate medical attention is required. Some signs of a severe reaction are blistered or burnt skin, difficulty breathing and a lot of swelling.

Oils that are known as "hot" oils have the ability to burn the skin in a manner similar to what happens with a chemical burn. Hot oils should never be applied directly to the skin at full strength. Some hot oils can be diluted with carrier oil and applied, but the risk of a reaction is higher when hot oils are used. Test them in a small area before applying them to a larger area of the body.

People who have health issues like diabetes, low or high blood pressure or any other medical condition should be aware that certain essential oils may worsen their condition and there are some essential oils that will dull or enhance the effects of certain medications. Additionally, some essential oils that are abortifacient or emmenagogue can bring about menstruation and cramping in women, so they need to be avoided when pregnant.

Because essential oils are powerful extracts, always consult with your physician before starting use of a new oil. There may be underlying health concerns you aren't aware of that he or she can call to your attention before you start taking the oil. It's also a good idea to consult with an aromatherapy practitioner to see what oils they recommend in light of your current physical condition. They may be able to tailor the oils you take to the health issues you currently have in order to help your body heal.

When trying out a new oil, it's critical you only use a small amount the first couple times. Even if the oil is generally regarded as safe, it's a good idea to dilute it heavily with carrier oil before the first application. Apply it and wait overnight to see if there's a reaction. If there's nothing wrong after 12 hours, you can try applying a little more oil. Watch your skin closely for signs of a reaction and discontinue use of the oil immediately if you suffer any ill effects.

There are a handful of essential oils that are too powerful to be used as part of an aromatherapy regime. Here are some of the oils you're going to want to steer clear of:

- **Alant root.**
- **Bitter almond.**
- **Boldo leaf.**
- **Calamus.**
- **Cassia.**
- **Horseradish.**
- **Mugwort.**
- **Mustard.**
- **Pennyroyal.**
- **Rue.**
- **Tansy.**
- **Thuja.**
- **Wintergreen.**
- **Wormwood.**
- **Yellow camphor.**

While you might see some resources that list health benefits associated with some of these oils, they aren't oils you should toy around with, especially if you don't know what you're doing. Some contain toxic substances and can make you sick or even kill you if they're used wrong. Keep in mind this isn't a complete list of all the oils that need to be avoided. It's just a sampling of some of the more toxic essential oils. These oils can cause everything from skin irritation to death, depending on the oil and how much of it is used.

The good news is you probably won't see most of these oils sold on store shelves in too many places. They're far too powerful for most manufacturers to sell to the general public.

What Makes Essential Oils So Powerful?

There are hundreds of natural chemical compounds that can exist in a single drop of essential oil. They combine in a variety of ways to give essential oils their individual fragrances and, arguably more importantly, their therapeutic qualities. The chemical composition of one essential oil can vary greatly in comparison to other oils, even amongst plants that seem similar at first glance.

Plants that have a similar smell like mint and peppermint may have some similarities when it comes to chemical composition, but no two plants will have the same blend. The chemical composition of essential oils can vary from plant to plant in different species and can be different amongst plants of the same species that are grown under varying conditions. That's why pure oils of the same type that come from different suppliers will have variances in scent and some may be far more effective than others when it comes to their therapeutic qualities. That's also the reason why lemons and limes smell similar, but you can tell the difference between them even though they're both citrus fruits and share a number of chemical compounds.

The therapeutic qualities of essential oils come about as a result of the individual chemical compounds entering the body and acting upon it in a number of ways. Each compound carries its own set of benefits and many of them act upon the body in ways scientists are just barely starting to grasp. It's important that you understand both the potential benefits and potential risks associated with any oil you want to use before you put it to use and that you have an understanding of the ways the oil could react when it enters your body.

The rest of this chapter discusses a number of the important compounds found in essential oils and their known effect on the human body.

Aldehydes

Aldehydes have strong fragrances and strong flavors. Cinnamon and vanilla both get their characteristic scents and flavors from aldehydes. The strong aroma of eucalyptus is also largely due to aldehydes. Other oils known to contain aldehydes include citronella, thyme and chamomile.

Oils containing these strong-scented compounds carry a number of therapeutic qualities, including the following:

- **Antibacterial.**
- **Antifungal.**
- **Anti-infectious.**
- **Anti-inflammatory.**
- **Antispasmodic.**
- **Antiviral.**
- **Aphrodisiac.**
- **Calming.**
- **Lower blood pressure.**
- **Relaxing.**
- **Sedative.**
- **Soothing.**
- **Stress relief.**
- **Tonic.**

Exercise care when using oils containing aldehydes, as they're dermal and mucous membrane irritants. This compound is one of the compounds that are responsible for allergic reactions to essential oils in sensitive individuals, so inhalation of the fragrances of oils containing aldehydes may be a better option than topical application. If you do decide to apply oils with aldehydes topically, dilute them heavily before application and always test them out in a small area first to see if there's a reaction. Tolerance to aldehydes varies from person to person, so never assume an oil is safe just because someone else didn't have a negative reaction to it.

Alcohols & Phenols

While drinking excessive amounts of alcohol can damage your inner workings, the alcohols found in essential oils are considered non-toxic and carry with them a number of benefits. They're antibacterial, antifungal, antiseptic, antiviral and are relatively stable in comparison to some of the other compounds found in essential oils. They're an immune stimulant and can be used to help soothe and heal damaged skin. They pass readily through the distillation process and are found in large amounts in oils like peppermint and geranium oil.

There are two basic types of alcohols found in essential oils. *Monoterpene alcohols* are the more common of the two and are relatively tame. Lavender, rose, tea tree and geranium oils all contain monoterpene alcohols in notable amounts. *Sesquiterpene alcohols* are less common, but carry some unique benefits with them when they're present. German chamomile contains a sesquiterpene alcohol known as bisabolol, which is thought to be a glandular stimulant that carries anti-allergy properties.

Phenols are another compound that is similar to alcohols. They're oxygenated molecules that are capable of cleansing cell receptors. They're said to carry the following properties:

- **Analgesic.**
- **Antibacterial.**
- **Anti-inflammatory.**
- **Antiseptic.**
- **Disinfectant.**
- **Oxygenating.**

- **Stimulant.**

Cinnamon, thyme and oregano oils all contain phenols. Exercise caution when using oils with phenols in them since they're a known dermal irritant. They're a powerful substance that can place a heavy load on the liver, so dilute them and only use small amounts. Extended use of oils with phenols in them isn't recommended.

Esters

Esters are created when alcohols react with acids in a process known as *esterification*. Essential oils that contain esters will usually have both alcohols and esters, but all of the acids in the oil will have been converted to esters. Esters are generally considered safe when they exist in essential oils.

They are known to carry the following the benefits:

- **Analgesic.**
- **Antifungal.**
- **Anti-inflammatory.**
- **Antispasmodic.**
- **Antiviral.**
- **Balancing.**
- **Calming.**
- **Sedative.**
- **Soothing.**
- **Uplifting.**

There are a number of essential oils that contain esters, including bergamot, lavender, clary sage, birch, myrrh, Roman chamomile and ylang ylang.

Ethers

Essential oils containing *ethers* are rare, but tend to be extremely powerful oils with strong scents and the potential to irritate the skin and mucous membranes. Some ethers are toxic in concentrated amounts and may have carcinogenic properties, so consult with a professional before using oils containing them.

Ketones

Unless you've been living under a rock, you've probably heard of raspberry ketones. They're hugely popular in the world of weight loss. What isn't as well-known is the fact that there are a number of other plants containing *ketones* and they're present in a small selection of essential oils.

Ketones are said to have the following benefits:

- **Antibacterial.**
- **Antifungal.**
- **Antispasmodic.**
- **Decongestant.**
- **Regenerative.**

Oils containing ketones usually only have small amounts of this powerful substance, but it still has a profound effect on the taste and fragrance of the plant. Some ketones like thujone are highly toxic and shouldn't be used by aromatherapy practitioners. Other ketones aren't as strong and can be used as long as you exercise caution. Camphor is found in basil, coriander, eucalyptus and rosemary oils. These oils can be diluted with carrier oils and applied externally as a decongestant that has a sedative effect on the person using it. They can also be used to relieve muscle pain in a manner similar to how you'd use Tiger Balm or Icy Hot.

Terpenes

The basic building block that most essential oils are made of is a molecule known as an *isoprene* that forms when 5 carbon atoms join in a row. *Terpenes* are created when isoprenes join together. When one isoprene molecule is present, it's known as a *hemiterpene*. Two isoprenes combined form a *monoterpene*, three form a *sesquiterpene* and four form a *diterpene*.

Monoterpenes contain 10 carbon atoms and exist in varying amounts in almost all essential oils. They're easily oxidized, which means oxygen atoms can bond to them to form other compounds, and they are easily damaged when heat is applied. Limonene is a common monoterpene that's found in citrus oils like grapefruit, lemon and lime. Pinene is another monoterpene that's found in pine, lavender and tea tree oil, amongst a number of other oils.

The benefits of monoterpenes vary widely depending on the type of monoterpene, but here are some of their more common properties:

- **Analgesic.**
- **Antibacterial.**
- **Anti-inflammatory.**
- **Antiseptic.**
- **Antiviral.**
- **Decongestant.**
- **Expectorant.**
- **Stimulant.**

Sesquiterpenes are made up of 15 carbon units and are less common. They have anti-inflammatory properties and oils containing them can sometimes be used to ward off allergies. Sandalwood, cedarwood and myrrh are all high in sesquiterpenes.

Sesquiterpenes are thought to have the following properties associated with them:

- **Analgesic.**
- **Antiallergic.**
- **Anti-inflammatory.**
- **Antiseptic.**
- **Hypotensive.**

Diterpenes contain 20 carbon atoms and are only found in significant amounts in a handful of essential oils. These heavy molecules may not make it through the distillation process if steam distillation is used because they're too heavy to evaporate. Diterpenes are believed to have the following properties:

- **Antifungal.**
- **Expectorant.**
- **Hormone balancing.**
- **Hypotensive.**

Terpenes make up a large amount of most essential oils, with some oils being made up of 70% or more terpenes. These compounds are the building blocks of essential oils and are responsible for the vast number of benefits they bestow upon people who use them. Without terpenes, essential oils wouldn't be anywhere near as effective as they are now.

Essential Oil Applications: How They're Used

There are three common methods used to apply essential oils to the body. Aromatherapy involves applying essential oils topically so that they're absorbed into the skin or by inhaling the aroma of the oils into the nose and lungs where they can be absorbed into the body. The third method of application is ingestion, which is beyond the scope of this book. While there are a handful of applications where ingestion of high-quality oil may be beneficial, there are also a number of inherent dangers and essential oils should not be consumed unless it's done under the supervision of a medical professional.

Certain oils lend themselves better to certain applications and applying an oil improperly can cause serious health problems. I'm not going to beat around the bush here. Even the weaker essential oils are very powerful concentrated essences and aren't something you should take lightly or play around with. Consuming or applying the wrong oil (or the wrong amount of the right oil) can be dangerous, so it's important you do your research carefully and exercise extreme caution.

Essential oils are at their best when they're diluted and are applied in tiny amounts. While a drop or two of essential oil mixed into a carrier oil may not seem like enough to make a difference, it helps to consider the fact it may have taken hundreds, if not thousands, of plants to fill the little vial of oil you're holding in your hand. Dilute your oils heavily before using them and be sure to test them out in small amounts before moving on to applying them to a larger area. You don't want to apply oil to your entire leg only to find out you're allergic to the particular essential oil or carrier oil you just applied. If that happens, you could be in for a world of hurt.

Inhaling the Fragrance of Essential Oils

Inhalation of essential oils is one of the most direct methods of internal application of essential oils. While you might think ingesting the oils would be faster, ingestion of the oils requires that they first pass through your digestive system where they're exposed to all sorts of acids and enzymes. It can take quite some time for the beneficial compounds to reach the blood stream, if they make it all. Ingestion of essential oils is rarely a good idea and there are a number of complications that can occur.

When you breathe in the fragrance of essential oils, you're breathing in tiny particles of the oil that are floating around in the air. That's why you're able to smell the oil when you inhale deeply. These tiny particles are absorbed into the soft tissues in your nasal cavity and lungs and are directly transferred into your blood stream. Additionally, they stimulate your olfactory nerve, which has a direct effect on your brain.

There are a number of ways essential oils can be forced into the air so they can be directly inhaled. Here are some of the easier methods:

- **Add a drop or two of oil to your hands,** place your hands around your nose and mouth and breathe deeply. Don't use this technique with "hot" oils that can burn the skin.
- **Add a drop or two of essential oil to a paper towel or handkerchief.** Hold the paper towel or handkerchief up to your nose and breathe the fragrance in.

- **Hold an open bottle of essential oil up to your nose and breathe in the fragrance.**
- **Soak a hand towel in warm water.** Wring it out and apply a few drops of essential oil to the towel. Let the towel cool enough to where it won't burn you and place it over your face. Breathe deeply.
- **Add several drops to the backside of your pillow.** Milder oils can be added to the front of your pillow, but be aware they may be transferred onto your face.

While it's a little more complicated, *diffusion* is a popular method of dispersing tiny droplets of essential oil into the air. With diffusion, essential oils are vaporized and dispersed into the around surrounding the vaporizer. This method allows you to fill a room with the fragrance of essential oils and everyone in the room will reap the benefits. You get the added benefit of the room smelling great while the oil is diffusing and being deodorized afterward.

There are two basic ways to diffuse essential oils: hot diffusion and cool diffusion. *Hot diffusion* uses a heat source to warm the essential oil up, causing it to evaporate.

Here are some of the more common hot diffusion methods:

- **Steam.** Essential oils are added to water and the water is heated up, causing it to evaporate.
- **Candle diffusers.** These diffusers place a candle below a well into which the essential oil is

placed. As the candle heats the well, the essential oil evaporates.

- **Wax warmers.** Essential oils are blended with wax. The warmers melt the wax and the oil is emitted into the room as the wax is heated to its melting point. Don't confuse this method with the wax fragrance blends from companies that use artificial fragrances like Scentsy. They smell good, but don't have the same benefits.
- **Electric diffusers.** These diffusers use either a heating element or a warm light bulb as a source of heat.

The problem with many of the hot methods of diffusing essential oils is the oils are sensitive to heat and can suffer damage as they're heated. The more heat that's used, the more damage the oil is likely to suffer. Use too much heat and you run the risk of changing the chemical structure of the oil and eliminating much of its potential health benefit. That hasn't stopped a large number of people from employing these methods, but many of them probably don't realize or don't care that applying heat can damage the oil. As long as their house smells good, they're happy!

If you're looking to reap the most reward from inhalation of essential oils, *cold diffusion* methods are the way to go. Instead of heating the oil, they use a number of innovative methods to break the oil up into small particles and disperse it into the room.

The following methods are all common ways of diffusing essential oils without using heat:

- **Cotton ball.** Add several drops of essential oil to a cotton ball and place it into a small bowl. Place the bowl in the middle of the room and the fragrance will quickly fill the room. This method works better in small rooms than it does in larger rooms.

- **Atomizers and nebulizers.** These machines break essential oils up into micro-particles that are dispersed into the room. Use these machines sparingly, as they can quickly fill a room with fine particles. Be aware that not all essential oils can be used in these machines.

- **Fans.** Some diffusers have small fans that blow air across the top of a reservoir into which you place essential oils.

- **Screen diffusers.** These diffusers push essential oils through fine-mesh screens that break them into tiny droplets that are then forced out into the room.

- **Reed diffusers.** This simple method places long wooden sticks into a pot of essential oils. The oils slowly make their way up the sticks and into the room.

- **Clay pots.** Terra cotta pots are made from a porous material. Oil is placed into the pots and it slowly seeps out, filling the room with its fragrance.

Keep in mind that some diffusion techniques disperse a lot of essential oil into a room in a short amount of time. These methods should be employed for a few minutes at a time and the diffuser should then be turned off until the scent of the oils no longer permeates the room.

Inhaling essential oils for a prolonged period of time can result in a condition known as *olfactory fatigue*. The human body is designed by nature to only smell new smells and it will quickly learn to ignore smells it's familiar with. This is a fight or flight response that stems from hundreds of thousands of years of having to use our senses to find food and to detect threats. If the brain determines a scent isn't food or some sort of danger, it puts it on the back burner and you'll stop noticing the smell. This is the reason people can live next to a garbage dump or a stinky cattle farm and seemingly go about their daily duties unaffected, but it makes us gag as soon as we're within smelling distance.

The fragrance of essential oils can be dismissed by the brain and you'll lose much of the calming and soothing effect of the oils. Olfactory fatigue can occur rather quickly, so it's best to expose yourself to 10- to 15-minute bursts of scent, as opposed to spending hours in a room into which essential oil has been dispersed. Spend too much time with a particular scent and the brain will almost become immune to it. You'll smell it right away when you first turn on the diffuser, but it'll be discarded quickly as a familiar scent that's neither food nor threat.

I have a small spare bedroom set up at my house that I use for diffusion. I go in there and have a seat in a comfy chair and read for 15 minutes while I enjoy my favorite oil blends. Once I'm done, I turn off the diffuser and leave the room. This allows me to enjoy the fragrance of the oils and reap the benefits of diffusion without having to worry about olfactory fatigue. In order to further combat this issue, I change the oil blends that I'm using at least once per week.

Applying Essential Oils to Your Skin

Topical application of essential oils involves applying them directly to your skin and rubbing them in. Most oils should be diluted first using what's known as a carrier oil, but there are a small handful of oils that can be applied neat.

Neat application simply means the oil is applied to the skin at full strength. There is more risk involved with neat application than diluted application because there are a number of oils known as "hot" oils that can burn the skin when applied neat. Additionally, the chances of your skin reacting negatively to an oil that isn't hot increases exponentially when it's applied neat. If you apply an essential oil neat and your body reacts negatively to it, you run the risk of not being able to use that oil anymore, even if it's diluted.

Because of the inherent risks associated with neat application, it's important this sort of treatment is done under the supervision of a professional. The only oil I ever apply neat is lavender oil and that's only because I've done it multiple times and have not had a reaction.

Most people are better served diluting essential oils with carrier oils before applying them to the skin. We'll cover carrier oils in detail later on in the book, but for now just realize they're weaker oils that are full of fats that are used to tone essential oils down so they aren't as powerful. A few drops of essential oil added to a tablespoon or more of carrier oil is all that's usually needed to reap the rewards of essential oils while minimizing the risk of a negative reaction.

Another method of direct application of essential oils is drawing a bath and adding them to the bath water. I've found it works best to add several drops of essential oil to the bath while the water is running because it helps disperse the oils into the bath. They'll eventually pool up on the top of the water and will coat your skin as you stand up when you're getting out of the tub. Be careful not to use the wrong type of oil (or too much of the right type of oil), as you have little control over how much is applied to your skin. A few drops in a full tub of water are usually all that's needed.

One more method that can be used is a warm compress. Run a sink full of warm water and add several drops of oil to the sink. Dip a towel or washcloth into the sink. Wring it out and hold it against your body in the area where you want to apply the oil. The warmth will open your pores and the oil will be able to enter your skin more easily than it otherwise would have. Don't use too hot of water or you run the risk of damaging the oils.

Carrier Oils: What They Are & How to Use Them

It's rarely a good idea to apply essential oils to the skin at full strength. This is especially true for "hot" oils because they have warming qualities and are more likely to burn the skin. When you apply an oil "neat," which means applying it at full strength, irritation similar to a minor chemical burn can occur. This irritation can permanently sensitize you to that oil.

Because of this risk, *carrier oils* are used to dilute essential oils before application. A carrier oil is a base oil that's fairly benign in regard to risk of skin reaction. Since most people can tolerate carrier oils, they're used to thin out essential oils and deliver them to the skin in a form that's easily tolerated. You still get the benefits of the oils, but the risk of irritation is greatly reduced.

Some carrier oils are used by themselves, but it's a more common for aromatherapy practitioners to blend them together. The oil blends they create can be perfectly suited to the skin type of the person they're going to be used on.

The amount of carrier oil that needs to be used in conjunction with an essential oil varies from oil to oil and can vary from person to person when using the same oil. It's going to take some experimentation to figure out the level at which you'll reap the most benefits without damaging your skin. Start off with a drop of essential oil mixed into a tablespoon of carrier oil and go from there. If it's well-tolerated, you might want to add a couple more drops the next time you use the oil. If there's a negative reaction, you should either use less essential oil the next time around or discontinue use of that oil.

Carrier oils are usually made up of nut or plant fats like coconut oil, almond oil or avocado oil, which come from coconut meat, almonds and avocadoes, respectively. Carrier oils are fatty oils that are usually pressed out of the fatty portions of the plant. They might slightly smell like the plant they were derived from, but they don't have the same strong fragrance that essential oils have. Organic cold-pressed carrier oils are generally considered the best for aromatherapy purposes. Steer clear of refined oils because they can contain trans fats and a number of harmful chemicals that make their way into the oil during refining.

A number of carrier oils are edible and are used in culinary recipes. Don't use carrier oils in recipes after you've added essential oils to them unless you're positive the oils are safe for consumption. Even then, you should be very careful and consult with your physician before adding essential oils to your diet.

In addition to making it less likely your skin will react negatively to essential oils, carrier oils also carry with them the following benefits:

- **Carrier oils get their name from their propensity to carry essential oils deep into the skin.**
- **Expensive essential oils are added to carrier oils in order to dilute the expensive oils while still realizing their benefits.** Carrier oils are

inexpensive and you can often buy large tubs for less than the cost of a small vial of essential oil.

- **Carrier oils sometimes have minor therapeutic benefits, including moisturizing and conditioning the skin.**
- **Carrier oils can be used to make natural skin care blends that can be rubbed into the skin.**
- **The amino acids in carrier oils are absorbed into the skin and make their way into your bloodstream.**

While some skin care recipes may call for mineral oil, steer clear of it when looking for an oil to combine with essential oils. Mineral oil is derived from petroleum and is anything but natural. You're much better off using natural carrier oils that won't clog your pores and block the essential oils from making their way into your body.

Apricot Kernel Oil

Apricot kernel oil is an inexpensive carrier oil that's pressed from apricot pits. It has a nutty fragrance with slightly fruity notes that are reminiscent of the apricots the oil was pressed from. It ranges in color from dark gold to translucent yellow. Apricot kernel oil is packed full of fatty acids, vitamins and minerals.

This oil is good for most skin types, but is especially well-suited to dry or aged skin. It moisturizes the skin and leaves an oily protective residue behind that helps lock moisture inside.

Avocado Oil

The sweet, nutty fragrance of avocado oil smells nothing like the fruit it comes from. The oil itself is a deep green color and is packed full of fatty acids, vitamins and minerals.

If you've got dry or damaged skin, avocado oil is a great choice. It heals and nourishes the skin while leaving behind a waxy protective coating. The after-feel of this oil takes some getting used to, but most people learn to love the benefits of avocado oil. It isn't usually used on its own. Instead, it's blended with other oils and is usually only around 10% of the overall oil blend.

It's another budget oil, so buying it to add to your oil blends won't break the bank.

Borage Seed Oil

Borage seed oil isn't cheap, but if you can afford the cost, it might be worth adding to your oil blends. The nice thing about this oil is it doesn't take much to reap the benefits associated with the high levels of gamma linoleic acid and you'll only need to use it as 10% of an oil blend.

Most skin types will benefit from use of borage seed oil, but it's especially beneficial for those with dry or damaged skin. The downside to using this oil is it leaves an oily residue behind that some people don't care for. It's one of the stronger carrier oils, so it shouldn't be used by pregnant women or people who are taking prescription medications without first consulting with their physician.

Castor Oil

Castor oil is pressed out of castor beans. It's another oil that shouldn't be used at full strength and is usually used as a 10% blend in oil blends. This oil has little to no scent, so it can be added to most oil blends with little effect on the overall fragrance. It's full of oleic acid and has a small amount of linoleic acid as well. It comes in various shades of translucent yellow and is a good choice for all skin types.

If you're looking for a carrier oil that will help disperse other oils into water, like when you're using essential oils in a bath or a spray bottle, castor oil is a great emulsifying agent that'll help spread the essential oils out into the bath water.

Coconut Oil

Coconut oil is one of the more popular carrier oils because of its cost and its ability to heal and tone the skin. It's a clear liquid when the temperature is warm, but will become a white solid as temperatures drop into the 70's. Pure coconut oil has a light, nutty smell with a faint hint of coconut.

It can be used without dilution, but you're better off mixing it into oil blends because it leaves behind an oily residue. While this residue isn't harmful, most people don't care for it, so they blend it with other less-greasy oils. Coconut oil can be used as a dispersant in oil blends you plan on adding to water.

Grapeseed Oil

Grapeseed oil is a great all-purpose oil that's inexpensive and easy to use. It can be used at full strength or you can use it in oil blends to take advantage of the high levels of linoleic acid it contains. It's derived from grape seeds, but instead of smelling like grapes, it has a light, nutty fragrance that dances around the nose.

If you're looking for an inexpensive carrier oil that's similar to some of the more costly oils, grapeseed oil is a good choice.

Jojoba Oil

This oil is derived from the fruit of the jojoba plant, which are fruits that aren't consumed by humans and are grown strictly for their oils. It's a mid-range priced oil with an aromatic fragrance that's unlike any other oil on the market. It melts into yellow liquid when the ambient temperature in the room is warm, but will solidify when temperatures start to cool off. Heat it up until it melts before adding it to oil blends.

Jojoba oil works best when blended into other oils at less than 10%. It's actually a liquid wax that's fairly close in consistency to the sebum that's emitted by the pores of the skin. It works best for oily and greasy skin types, but will work for pretty much any other skin type as well.

Macadamia Nut Oil

Macadamia nut oil has a strong nutty aroma that's overpowering at full strength, so it's usually blended as 10% or less of an oil blend. Another good reason to blend it is the fact that it's thick and will leave an oily sheen on your skin. Pure macadamia nut oil is clear with a slight hint of yellow.

If you've got sensitive skin, macadamia nut oil might be a good choice due to its high oleic acid content.

Olive Oil

If you've ever smelled olive oil that's used for cooking, you know what olive oil smells like. It has the moderately-strong aroma of olives and should be diluted heavily as part of an oil blend if you want to use it.

Because of its smell and the thick viscosity of the oil, olive oil isn't a popular choice for aromatherapy. It's also been known to cause skin reactions in sensitive individuals. Unless it's all you have, the other oils in this chapter are usually much better options.

Rosehip Seed Oil

At a price point of around $30 for 4 ounces of organic oil, rosehip seed oil falls on the more expensive side of the spectrum. Luckily, it doesn't take much of this oil to add a hefty amount of fatty acids to your oil blend. This oil is usually blended at 10% dilution or less.

It has a mild aroma that smells nothing like the rose hips it was obtained from. It only leaves a light residue and is one of the more desirable oils for those with naturally-oily skin. Buy this oil in small amounts and use it up quickly. It can go rancid within 6 months of opening the bottle.

Sesame Oil

This inexpensive option is pressed from sesame seeds, and while it's a good choice for most skin types, it's especially effective for those with psoriasis or eczema because it's packed full of oleic and linoleic acids. It has a sweet, nutty aroma that melds well with most essential oils. Sesame seed oil is translucent yellow in color and leaves behind a protective sheen.

Dilute it to 10% or less of an oil blend or you run the risk of overpowering the scent of the essential oils in the blend.

Sunflower Seed Oil

Sunflower seed oil is one of the few carrier oils that don't leave behind an oily sheen. It penetrates into the skin and carries essential oils deep below the surface, leaving little behind. It's an affordable oil and is a good choice for most aromatherapy purposes, as long as you're using unrefined oil. The slightly sweet aroma isn't overpowering, so sesame seed oil is often used at full strength or as a base oil for oil blends.

Sunflower seed oil comes in two forms. The standard form is packed with linoleic acids, while the High Oleic Acid form tilts the balance toward oleic acid.

Sweet Almond Oil

Sweet almond oil has a sweet, slightly nutty fragrance and is one of the less-expensive carrier oils. It's pressed out of almond kernels and is a translucent yellow color when it's in its purest form. While it's a popular choice amongst those who are looking for a budget oil that's full of fatty acids, it can cause allergic reactions in those who are allergic to nuts.

It's a good choice for most skin types and will soften and condition skin that it's rubbed into. Some people don't care for the light oily residue it leaves behind, but it helps to think of the residue as a protective coating that shields the skin.

Watermelon Seed Oil

Watermelon seed oil is another good base oil that can be blended with other oils to create oil blends. It has a slightly nutty fragrance that isn't overpowering, so it's often the main oil in the blends it's added to. This oil is thin and penetrates well, leaving a very slight oily sheen in its wake.

This oil is a good choice for all skin types, but is particularly effective on oily skin.

How to Find High Quality Essential Oils

Finding essential oils that are of high quality isn't easy because there are no set standards by which essential oils are judged. The government doesn't control the standards to which essential oils are held and there is no set governing body, so it's up to the individual to determine which oils are of good quality and which oils aren't. This can be difficult because quality can vary from company to company and from oil to oil within a company and the consumer ends up having to decipher all sorts of marketing terms used to sell oils that may or may not mean something in the grand scheme of things.

You'll see manufacturers that claim their oil is "therapeutic" or "essential oil" grade or some other marketing term they've created to try to sell more oil. While the oil they sell may be good oil, it's important to judge the oils based on their individual attributes and not some term made up by a marketing department. Avoid oils that are labeled as food grade or perfume grade because they may not be up to the standards required for aromatherapy.

There are a lot of considerations that must be made when choosing a brand of essential oils, including the following:

- **The type of plants used and where they're grown.** Different varieties of plants may produce varying qualities of oils. Plants grown under optimal conditions will produce oils that are of higher quality than those produced by stressed plants growing in less-than-optimal conditions.

- **The altitude at which the plants are grown.** If plants are grown at too high or too low of an altitude, the quality of the essential oil can be impacted.

- **Organically-grown plants.** Oil that comes from organically-grown plants is less likely to contain trace amounts of the pesticides and other chemicals that conventionally-grown plants are treated with.

- **Harvest and storage.** The essential oils contained within plant matter will begin to degrade shortly after the plant is harvested. The best essential oils are extracted from plants shortly after they're harvested.

- **The part of the plant that's used.** Oil can be extracted from all parts of a plant. Oil pulled from seeds will differ from oil pulled from stems, which will differ from oil pulled from flowers.

- **The extraction method used.** The method that's used to pull the oil out of the plant will impact the final quality of the oil. Steam distillation can damage heat-sensitive compounds in some oils and may leave heavier compounds behind. Solvent-extraction is the least-desirable extraction method because trace amounts of the chemical solvent will end up in the oil. This puts the consumer at odds with some manufacturers because solvent-extraction is often the most cost-effective form of extraction.

- **Additives.** Don't use oils that have additives, if at all possible. Some of the more expensive oils are diluted with other oils to bring down the price and make them more accessible to the average person. This is fine, but be aware that some companies have been known to dilute expensive oils without labeling them.

The best oils are pure, unadulterated oils that are extracted using methods that don't damage the oil and don't add anything to it. The problem lies in the lack of transparency on the parts of the oil manufacturers. This information isn't always readily available and you may have to contact the manufacturer directly to get a clear answer. Even then, there's no guarantee you're going to get the truth.

I typically stick to trusted brands and avoid the cut-rate manufacturers out there that are selling essential oils for rock-bottom prices. I don't mind paying a little bit extra for quality oils that were extracted using safe methods. Once you're familiar with the going rate for good oils, it isn't hard to spot a company that's probably not selling good oil based on their low prices alone.

Here are a handful of companies that are generally trusted by their customers and are thought to produce good essential oils:

http://www.100pureessentialoils.com/

http://www.amphora-retail.com/
http://www.aqua-oleum.co.uk/
http://www.aromaticsinternational.com/
http://www.auroma.com/
http://www.camdengrey.com/
http://www.e-scent-ials.com/
http://www.fromnaturewithlove.com
http://www.gardenofessence.com/#!store
http://www.mountainroseherbs.com
http://www.doterra.com/
http://ww.youngliving.com/

Keep in mind the last two companies on the list, DoTerra and Young Living are MLM companies and may try to sign you up to sell their oils when you attempt to make a purchase. I don't personally use oils from either of those companies at this point in time, but I've tried them in the past and have found them to be of good quality.

Another consideration you should make is there is no single company that makes the best essential oils. I've found the quality of individual oils varies within a company, so I buy different oils from different companies. If I purchase an oil from a company and I like it, I'll continue buying that oil. If I buy other types of oil from that company and they aren't up to my standards, I'll try different companies for the other oils until I find one I like.

Essential oils are becoming more and more popular and I've been seeing them pop up in big-box retailers and health food stores. The oils I've seen in these stores so far have been budget oils and the oils I've tried haven't been of good quality. If all you want to do is make a room in your house smell good, these oils might get the job done, but they probably don't carry the same therapeutic qualities as the better oils have.

When searching for a company to buy essential oils from, you generally get what you pay for. Rock-bottom prices for essential oils is almost always an indicator of sub-par oils or oils that have been adulterated with other compounds. If you find an oil you want at a price that's too good to be true, research the company you're considering buying the oil from before making a purchase. You might be surprised (or not so surprised after reading this book) to find the company has a poor reputation and/or sells oils that aren't what they claim they are.

When purchasing essential oils, you're going to find some oils cost a small fortune, while others are relatively inexpensive. This is because some oils are extremely difficult to extract and take a lot of plants to obtain a small amount of oil. Take rose otto oil for example. At $400 per ounce, it's one of the more expensive oils, but the cost is so high because it takes a couple dozen roses to produce a single drop of oil. If you see this oil at a price that seems too good to be true, be very cautious. The companies selling these oils at low prices are probably selling oil that's been adulterated and the oil inside may not be rose otto oil at all.

Are the Oils You're Buying Sustainable?

While sustainability won't affect the quality of the oils you're buying, it does affect the quality of the Earth, the health of the ecosystem where the plants the oils are extracted from are grown and it negatively impacts many of the people who live in the area where the plants are farmed. Most essential oils come from farming operations in foreign countries where the methods used to grow and/or harvest the essential oils aren't heavily regulated. Even when they are regulated, there are unscrupulous oil companies that are willing to do whatever it takes to get their oils at an acceptable price.

It's easy for consumers to turn a blind eye to sustainability because unsustainable harvesting of plants lowers the costs of essential oils in the short term. While there are plenty of plants available for the taking, mass harvesting of these plants makes it so the oils are available in large amounts and prices go down. It'll eventually catch up to all of us and the costs of oils like sandalwood, which is harvested from the heartwood of trees that need to grow for decades before oil can be harvested from them, will shoot up as there are fewer and fewer harvestable trees available. Wild-harvested oils that come from herbs or spices can also be problematic as far as sustainability. These oils aren't farmed, so in order to obtain them the oil producer has to clear large swaths of wild growth.

Before buying any essential oil, it's important to research where that oil came from and how it's harvested.

Failure to properly vet where your oils came from may result in you unknowingly assisting those who are destroying the environment just to make a quick buck. The company you buy your essential oils from should be able to tell you where they came from and how they're harvested. If they can't tell you (or they seem unwilling to do so), there's usually a reason they're keeping quiet. Move on to another manufacturer who's more transparent about where their oil comes from.

The Essential Oils Guide

There I was, new to the world of essential oils, standing in front of shelf after shelf packed full of bottles of essential oils. I'd heard they were good to use for a number of therapeutic applications, but I didn't know much more than that. As I scanned the labels, I realized I was in way over my head. Tea tree oil, eucalyptus oil, lavender oil. I recognized the names of some of the plants the oils came from, but really had no clue what the oils were for.

I grabbed a couple oils that I thought sounded interesting and headed home with them. In hindsight, I'm very lucky I grabbed lavender oil and tea tree oil because they're on the milder side of the spectrum. Had I have grabbed one of the hotter oils, my first essential oil experience might not have gone so well.

This guide doesn't contain every essential oil out there. Instead, it seeks to give you enough information on the more popular essential oils sold today to where you can make an informed decision as to which oils you want to purchase. I really could have used a guide like this when I was just starting out and I'm sure there are plenty of others who could as well.

You obviously aren't going to buy every essential oil out there. Nobody I know has them all. Instead, you're going to want to buy a handful of oils you think are best-suited to your individual needs. Some might work great, others not-so-much. It's a learning process and each person's body reacts differently to different oils. Discard the ones that don't work well (or give them away) and continue gradually buying and testing oils until you've got a collection that's perfectly suited to your individual needs.

Essential Oil Terminology

Unless you've been around essential oils for a while and are well-studied, you're going to come across a number of terms you might not be familiar with as you go through the rest of the book. If you see a term describing a quality an oil has that you aren't familiar with, check here to see what it means.

Abortifacient

May cause contractions and induce abortion. Don't use oils labeled as being abortifacient if you're pregnant or are attempting to get pregnant. This should go without saying, but you shouldn't use them to attempt an abortion either. These oils don't always cause abortion, but may cause irreversible damage to an unborn fetus.

Alopecia

A form of baldness.

Analgesic

Able to cause numbness or relieve minor pain.

Anesthetic

Similar to analgesic. Relieves pain by deadening the area it's applied to.

Antacid

Helps quell the effects of stomach acid.

Antiarthritic

Able to help quell the effects of arthritis. May provide minor pain relief.

Antiallergenic

Able to reduce the symptoms caused by allergies. Don't use these oils to attempt to treat food allergies.

Antibacterial

Able to kill or combat harmful bacteria.

Antibiotic

Similar to antibacterial. Antibiotics fight bacteria inside the body.

Anticonvulsant

May be able to aid with the control of convulsions.

Antidepressant

Fights depression by improving your mood.

Antidontalgic

Relieves the pain associated with toothaches.

Antifungal

Quells the growth of fungi.

Antigalactagogue

Slows the flow of milk in nursing women. Depending on whether or not you're breast feeding, this effect may or may not be desirable.

Antihemorrhagic

Slows bleeding.

Antihistamine

Able to combat an allergic reaction by blocking histamine receptors from reacting to the compounds causing the reaction.

Anti-infectious

Helps the body fight off infection.

Anti-inflammatory

Helps reduce inflammation.

Antimicrobial

Kills or reduces the impact of microbes.

Antioxidant

Helps prevent oxidation and promotes better health on a cellular level.

Antiparasitic

Fights off parasites.

Antipruritic

Provides itch relief.

Antipyretic

Helps the body fight off fever.

Antirheumatic

Fights off the symptoms of rheumatism.

Antiseborrheic

Great for oily skin. Helps the body control the release of sebum from skin pores.

Antiseptic

Helps control infection.

Antispasmodic

Prevents or lessens the severity of spasms.

Antisudorific

Reduces the amount of moisture released while sweating.

Aperient

Has mild laxative qualities.

Aphrodisiac

Has the ability to cause sexual arousal.

Astringent

Causes tissue to contract. Oils that have this quality may make the skin feel taut when they're applied.

Bactericidal

Eliminates bacteria on contact.

Carcinogenic

Can cause cancer and may promote the growth of tumors. Avoid carcinogenic oils at all costs.

Carminative

Relieves flatulence and soothes the stomach.

Cholagogue

Promotes the discharge of bile.

Cicatrisant

Promotes healing through the formation of scar tissue. To be clear, this quality causes scar tissue to grow to promote faster healing. It doesn't help get rid of scar tissue that's already present.

Decongestant

Helps relieve congestion and clear up mucus.

Depurative

Purifying

Diuretic

Promotes urine flow and helps remove water and toxins from the body.

Emmenagogue

Brings on menstruation. Do not use oils with emmenagogue properties while pregnant or when attempting to get pregnant.

Emollient

Smooths and softens the skin.

Expectorant

Helps remove mucus from the lungs.

Febrifuge

Fights fever.

Galactagogue

Encourages milk production.

Hemostatic

Slows or stops bleeding.

Laxative

Brings on bowel movement.

Lipolytic

Causes the body to eliminate fats.

Mucolytic

Breaks mucus down and dispels it.

Narcotic

Brings on sleep and drowsiness.

Nervine

Makes the immune system stronger.

Prophylactic

Helps prevent disease.

Rubefacient

Causes redness of the skin due to increased blood flow near the surface.

Stomachic

Helps ease stomach issues and aids with digestion.

Sudorific

Causes sweating.

Vermifuge

Eliminates intestinal worms.

Vulnerary

Heals wounds.

Allspice Oil

Allspice oil isn't the most popular essential oil around, but it's a great all-around oil that has a number of benefits. I recommend allspice oil as the first essential oil you buy and use, but once you've got a nice collection going it's a good oil to have on hand. It isn't cheap, but it isn't going to break the bank either.

The leaves and fruit of the allspice, or pimento, tree contain most of the oil. It has a spicy, sweet fragrance with hints of cinnamon and cloves that blends well with most oils, but works particularly well when blended with geranium, lavender, patchouli or ylang ylang oil.

The following properties are associated with allspice oil:

- **Analgesic.**
- **Anesthetic.**
- **Antibacterial.**
- **Antifungal.**
- **Antioxidant.**
- **Antiseptic.**
- **Antiviral.**
- **Aphrodisiac.**
- **Carminative.**
- **Muscle relaxer.**
- **Rubefacient.**
- **Stimulant.**
- **Tonic.**

I prefer vaporizing allspice oil over applying it to the skin, however when I have a cold and am feeling congested, I do like to add a drop or two of allspice oil to a tablespoon of carrier oil and rub it into my chest. The warming properties of allspice oil make it a good choice for use on aches and pains and muscle spasms. Diffusing allspice can help relieve stress and may even pull you out of a funk if you're feeling down. It relieves tension and anxiety, so it can be used to unwind after a long day.

The eugenol, menthyl eugnenol and ceneol found in allspice oil contribute to its warming properties. It's considered a hot oil that should always be diluted before it's applied. The risk of dermal or mucus membrane irritation is fairly high, so always test it in small amounts in an inconspicuous area prior to application over a broader area. It needs to be diluted even when it's diffused because diffusing it at full strength can cause mucous membrane irritation when it's inhaled. Do not use allspice oil if pregnant.

Basil Oil

If you've ever cooked with basil, you know what basil essential oil smells like, except the oil is in a much more concentrated form and the smell is stronger. It has a light, peppery scent that's stronger than smelling a sprig of fresh basil, but isn't overwhelmingly strong. Basil essential oil is extracted from the leaves and flowers of the basil plant. Steam distillation is the most common method used to obtain basil oil.

Basil oil has the following properties:

- **Antibacterial.**
- **Antidepressant.**
- **Antiseptic.**
- **Antispasmodic.**
- **Carminative.**
- **Expectorant.**
- **Stimulant.**
- **Tonic.**

The fragrance of basil oil has a stimulating effect on most people, waking them up and leaving them feeling refreshed, but for some the effect can be the opposite. It makes a small percentage of the people who use it drowsy and will visibly slow them down. If you try basil oil and you're one of those people, don't use basil oil in the mornings. Instead, wait until the evenings and use it as a natural sleep aid. On the other hand, if you fall squarely in the group that's stimulated by basil oil, don't use it in the evening or you may have trouble falling asleep.

Basil oil works well to help relieve the effects of the common cold. When I diffuse basil oil into a room when I'm sick, it clears up congestion and helps bring me out of the brain fog I'm in. I've also used it to relieve aches and pains associated with both the common cold and the flu and have used it from time to time when I had stubborn headaches that wouldn't go away.

Those who are epileptic should avoid basil oil. Pregnant women should avoid it as well and it shouldn't be used on children under the age of 16. This oil is strong, so there's some risk of skin irritation. Always dilute basil oil before topical application and test it in a small area. A couple drops of basil oil mixed into a teaspoon of carrier oil is all that's needed to get the full effect. It's a good idea to contact the supplier you're planning on buying basil oil from to check to see how much methyl chavicol the basil oil contains. This substance occurs naturally in basil oil and is a suspected carcinogen. Because of the risks associated with methyl chavicol, basil oil should only be used occasionally and always in small amounts.

I prefer blending basil oil to using it alone. It blends well with cedarwood, citrus oils, citronella, clary sage and rosemary, but you have to be careful not to use too much or all you'll be able to smell is the basil oil.

Bergamot Oil

Bergamot oil comes from the fruit of the *Citrus bergamia* plant, which is a citrus fruit that is the size and shape of an orange, but is yellow like a lemon. It's grown commercially along the Ivory Coast, in southern France and in Southern Italy. Bergamot fruit isn't consumed as a food item, but the locals will juice it and drink the bitter juice. It's also made into marmalade.

Bergamot essential oil is extracted from the peel of the plant. It's dark to light green in color and is a mixture of esters, terpenes, alcohols and aldehydes. It has a light citrus fragrance with floral notes that dance around your nose, making it a popular choice for perfumes and natural bath and body products. This essential oil is one that's commonly adulterated, so make sure you purchase it from a reputable supplier.

The following properties have been associated with bergamot oil:

- **Analgesic.**
- **Antibiotic.**
- **Antidepressant.**
- **Antiseptic.**
- **Antispasmodic.**
- **Astringent.**
- **Calming.**
- **Deodorant.**

Since bergamot oil is astringent, it can be used in place of a number of over-the-counter acne treatments. It works well for people who have oily skin and are looking to clear it up. Start with a drop or two added to coconut oil and work your way up from there until you find the right blend for your skin type.

Diffuse bergamot oil into a room or inhale it directly and you'll instantly feel calm and relaxed. A great use for bergamot oil is to blend it with lavender and use it to wind down after a rough day. It can also be used to help fight off sadness on those days you're feeling a little blue and to relieve stress when the world gets to be too much to handle. I've heard of people using it to fight off anxiety and fears as well.

Be aware bergamot oil has been shown to cause sensitivity to ultraviolet light. Don't apply it to areas of skin that are going to be exposed to the sun or they may become red and irritated. Bergaptene is the compound in the oil that's responsible for this reaction. Some manufacturers offer bergamot oil that's low in bergaptene, but it can still cause a reaction in those with sensitive skin. It can also be a dermal irritant at full strength, so be sure to dilute it with carrier oil before topical application.

Bergamot oil has a light fragrance that blends well with most essential oils. Some of the oils it melds well with include chamomile, other citrus oils, geranium, jasmine, juniper, lavender, lemon balm, rose, sandalwood and ylang ylang oil.

Cardamom Seed Oil

Cardamom seed oil comes from the seeds of the cardamom plant, which you may be familiar with as a cooking spice. The scientific name of the cardamom plant is *Elettaria cardamomum*. The oil is extracted from the seeds and is translucent in color with a light yellow tint. It has a sweet, spicy fragrance that isn't unlike what the cooking spice smells like.

This interesting oil has the following benefits associated with it:

- **Antibacterial.**
- **Anti-infectious.**
- **Anti-inflammatory.**
- **Antimicrobial.**
- **Antiseptic.**
- **Antispasmodic.**
- **Aphrodisiac.**
- **Decongestant.**
- **Digestive.**
- **Diuretic.**
- **Energizing.**
- **Expectorant.**
- **Stimulant.**
- **Stomachic.**
- **Stomachic.**
- **Uplifting.**

The most common use of cardamom oil is as a digestive aid and to help promote good respiratory health. It isn't as strong as other oils like eucalyptus and peppermint that are typically used to help battle respiratory infections, but is just as effective in its own right. Start by diffusing cardamom oil or inhaling steam containing cardamom oil and if that doesn't work, then it might be time to break out the big guns and use peppermint or eucalyptus oil.

Cardamom oil ranks amongst the top sellers when it comes to people looking for an essential oil with aphrodisiac qualities. It's also said to aid with impotence and may promote a more rapid sexual response.

When feelings of anger are starting to consume you, cardamom oil can be used to bring you back down to earth. It's uplifting and energizing and you may find the items you were angry about really weren't that big of a deal once you've had a chance to step back and reexamine them.

Cardamom oil can be diffused on its own, but is more-commonly added to oil blends to up their effectiveness. Most people are able to tolerate neat application, but it's a warming oil and many prefer adding a few drops to an oil blend and diluting it with carrier oil before applying it topically. Be careful not to use too much cardamom oil. It can cause profuse sweating and may cause feelings of unrest. Pregnant women and breastfeeding mothers should avoid using this oil.

Floral oils and wood oils are good choices for blending with cardamom oil.

Cedarwood Oil

Cedarwood oil is extracted from the wood and roots of cedar trees. It's one of the oldest oils known to man and has been in use since the days of the ancient Egyptians when it was used for mummification and to repel insects. If you've ever smelled a cedar chest, the fragrance of the oil is similar. It has a clean, woodsy smell that reminds me of a number-2 pencil and is pale to light yellow in color.

The following therapeutic properties have been associated with cedarwood oil:

- **Antifungal.**
- **Antiseborrheic.**
- **Antiseptic.**
- **Antispasmodic.**
- **Astringent.**
- **Diuretic.**
- **Emmenagogue.**
- **Expectorant.**
- **Insect repellent.**
- **Sedative.**
- **Tonic.**

This woodsy oil is astringent, so it benefits oily skin and is good for acne. It can also be used as a remedy for dandruff and oily hair. Combine it with rosemary oil and rub it into your scalp to help prevent alopecia or hair loss. The most common use of cedarwood oil in aromatherapy is for respiratory health. It can be rubbed into the chest to ease the effects of asthma and a couple drops can be applied to the throat or neck to help clear up congestion.

The sedative effects of cedarwood oil can be realized through inhalation or by diluting the oil with carrier oil and applying it topically. It can be used to calm overanxious people down and to relieve nervous tension. It's said to help ground people and may invoke feelings of confidence and self-worth. It's also said to act as an aphrodisiac.

Another great use for cedarwood oil is as an insect repellant. Dilute it with carrier oil and apply it topically to keep bugs at bay while you're out and about or diffuse it into an area of your home where you want to get rid of insects. I use it during the summer to keep the flies out of my kitchen and I've been known to add a few drops here and there to my screened porch to keep the insects away while I'm hanging out sipping tea on summer evenings. A drop or two on your pet's collar can be used to keep fleas and ticks at bay.

Cedarwood oil can irritate the skin when large amounts are used, so exercise caution. Pregnant women should avoid use of this oil. It blends well with citrus oils, other wood oils, frankincense, jasmine and rose oil. Citrus oils are my favorite because they take the bite associated with the scent of cedarwood away and make it more tolerable.

Chamomile, German

German chamomile, also known as blue chamomile or wild chamomile, comes from the *Matricaria recutita* plant and is a deep blue oil that's steam-distilled from the flowers of the chamomile plants it's extracted from. It gets its blue color from a chemical known as chamazulene, which has strong anti-inflammatory properties.

Don't confuse German chamomile with Roman chamomile. They both come from plants from the same family, but are remarkably different essential oils. German chamomile essential oil has a sweet, herbaceous aroma, while Roman chamomile has a light, fruity fragrance with hints of apple. Roman chamomile doesn't contain the high levels of chamazulene that German chamomile features.

German chamomile has the following properties:

- **Analgesic.**
- **Antiallergenic.**
- **Antibacterial.**
- **Antibiotic.**
- **Anti-inflammatory.**
- **Antispasmodic.**
- **Carminative.**
- **Cholagogue.**
- **Cicatrisant.**
- **Emmenagogue.**
- **Hepatic.**
- **Sedative.**
- **Stomachic.**
- **Vermifuge.**

- **Vulnerary.**

The anti-inflammatory properties of German chamomile are strong, so it can be used to calm both internal and external inflammation. Dilute it with carrier oil and rub it on the inflamed area for relief. It works well on skin problems like dry, flaky skin and skin damaged by acne, psoriasis and eczema The emmenagogue properties of German chamomile helps to promote menstrual flow and it may provide at least some relief for women going through menopause. Combine it with clary sage oil to up its effectiveness. It's also good for allergy relief and may provide relief from headaches and migraines.

Diffuse German chamomile into a room to calm frayed nerves and soothe the soul. It levels out hot emotions like anger and frustration and replaces them with peacefulness and clarity of mind. If you're looking for answers to a problem, but can't see past your raw emotion, German chamomile may help set you on the right path.

German chamomile is generally thought to be nontoxic and can be used by most people without irritation. It does have emmenagogue properties and shouldn't be used by pregnant women.

Many people opt to use German chamomile by itself, but it can also be blended with other oils. Bergamot, clary sage, lavender, tea tree and ylang ylang oil are all oils it's commonly blended with.

Chamomile, Roman

Roman chamomile oil comes from the *Chamaemeleum nobile* plant. Don't get this oil confused with German chamomile, which comes from a similar, but different plant. Also be aware that some companies try to substitute *Ormenis multicaulis* for *Chamaemeleum nobile*. The two plants are not the same, so avoid Roman chamomile made from any plant other than *Chamaemeleum nobile*.

Roman chamomile has a fruity, herbaceous fragrance that calms and soothes the mind, body and soul. Its middle notes are reminiscent of apple, giving it a light, refreshing aroma. It can be diffused, inhaled directly or applied topically, but should be diluted before topical application because it's a somewhat warm oil and there's a slight risk of skin irritation if it's applied neat. Internal consumption isn't recommended for most brands.

This oil is said to have the following properties:

- **Analgesic.**
- **Antiallergenic.**
- **Antibacterial.**
- **Antibiotic.**
- **Antidepressant.**
- **Anti-inflammatory.**
- **Antimicrobial.**
- **Antiparasitic.**
- **Antiseptic.**
- **Antispasmodic.**
- **Calming.**
- **Carminative.**

- **Cholagogue.**
- **Emmenagogue.**
- **Febrifuge.**
- **Heals the skin.**
- **Sedative.**
- **Stomachic.**
- **Sudorific.**
- **Tonic.**

It's believed to uplift your spirit and may be able to help those who are feeling purposeless or discouraged come to grips with where they're at in life. If you suffer from insomnia, inhaling this oil at bed time or diffusing it into the room you're planning on sleeping in may help you relax and drift off to sleep.

Add a few drops of Roman chamomile to a tablespoon of carrier oil and rub it into dry, irritated areas of your skin for almost-instant relief. It penetrates deep below the surface of the skin, so it can also be used to sooth minor aches and pains and is commonly used by those looking to ease arthritis pain. One of my favorite uses of this oil is to combine it with lavender oil and coconut oil and rub it into sore muscles after I work out.

Most sources indicate Roman chamomile is safe for older children, which is good because it soothes sunburns, bug bites, scrapes and mild burns and promotes faster healing. Don't apply it to open cuts or wounds. It works great when applied to bee stings and will ease the pain on contact.

If you or a loved one suffers from seasonal allergies, try diffusing this oil into the house daily as soon as you first feel your allergies start to flare up. Alternatively, dilute Roman chamomile with carrier oil and rub it into your feet and hands regularly. It can also be inhaled directly to provide relief when allergies get particularly troublesome.

This handy oil also works great on animals. It can be used to calm nervous dogs and horses. Certain oils can be toxic to cats, so consult with your vet before applying it to your cat.

If you're looking to blend this oil with other oils, there are a number of good choices. Bergamot, clary sage, eucalyptus, citrus oils, lavender, rose and tea tree oil are all good choices.

While this is a commonly-used essential oil, there are some safety considerations that should be made. It's considered non-toxic, but shouldn't be used by pregnant women or people who are allergic to ragweed because the plant it comes from is in a similar family.

Cinnamon Oil

Cinnamon essential oil is distilled from either the leaves or the bark of the *Cinnamomum zeylanicum* plant. Cinnamon bark oil will typically cost more than cinnamon leaf oil because it's more difficult to distill oil from bark than it is to get it out of the leaves. Both oils have the strong aroma of cinnamon, but the oil from the leaves contains elevated levels of eugenol and may smell more like cloves than cinnamon. Pure cinnamon oil will be dark yellow to brown in color and feel oily to the touch.

Since it smells similar to the cinnamon used to flavor culinary dishes, people often assume the oil comes from the same plant, but that assumption is incorrect. Most of the cinnamon sold in stores today is actually cassia, which is a different plant. There is cassia essential oil that smells strongly of cinnamon, but it should be avoided because of its toxicity.

Both cinnamon leaf and cinnamon bark oil can be dermal irritants and should not be applied directly to the skin. Cinnamon bark oil is stronger than cinnamon leaf oil and may be more hazardous. For this reason, cinnamon bark oil isn't usually used for aromatherapy purposes and should probably be avoided in favor of cinnamon leaf oil. The rest of this chapter discusses the potential uses of cinnamon leaf oil.

Cinnamon leaf oil has a number of therapeutic qualities that have been associated with it, including the following:

- **Analgesic.**
- **Antibacterial.**
- **Antifungal.**

- **Anti-inflammatory.**
- **Antimicrobial.**
- **Antirheumatic.**
- **Antiseptic.**
- **Antispasmodic.**
- **Aphrodisiac.**
- **Astringent.**
- **Carminative.**
- **Emmenagogue.**
- **Expectorant.**
- **Insecticide.**
- **Stimulant.**
- **Stomachic.**
- **Tonic.**
- **Vermifuge.**

Because of the risk of dermal irritation, the preferred method of use for cinnamon leaf oil is diffusion. However, it can be heavily diluted with carrier oil and massaged into the skin. Make sure you test the oil in a small area prior to applying it to larger areas of the body. Avoid use of cinnamon oil if you're pregnant or are attempting to get pregnant.

Cinnamon leaf oil works well for minor respiratory issues and has seen some use for respiratory conditions like bronchitis and coughs associated with flus or colds. It can also be used to ease muscle and joint pain and its analgesic properties may provide some relief from the pain associated with arthritis, rheumatism or gout. Those with athlete's foot can add a couple drops of cinnamon leaf oil to a tub of warm water and soak their feet in it.

Diffused cinnamon leaf oil acts as a mild antidepressant and may help improve your mood. It's thought to improve cognitive function and may improve mental acuity. When you're feeling down in the dumps, diffusing this oil may be all you need to turn your mood around and start feeling better.

Add 10 to 20 drops of cinnamon leaf oil to a spray bottle full of water and shake it up to create a homemade cleaner that has disinfectant properties and will fill your home with the warm smell of cinnamon. Use it on cutting boards or spray it inside your fridge to stop foul odors dead in their tracks. It can also be used on toilets, dishwashers and any other hard surface you want to disinfect. I've even seen it sprayed inside tennis shoes to refresh them and eliminate foul odors.

The homemade cleaner can also be used as an insect repellent that will repel and possibly even kill insects ranging from house ants to flies. It's also a great deterrent for roaches, but you've got to use it regularly to keep them at bay. Cinnamon leaf oil can even be used as a deterrent for bed bugs. Spray it on mattresses and other area where bed bugs tend to congregate and let it dry to keep bed bugs out of your bedroom. Be aware that cinnamon oils might stain lighter colored sheets and mattresses when applied frequently.

Cinnamon leaf oil can be used as the sole oil in a blend, but it really comes into its own when combined with other essential oils. It blends well with citrus oils, clove oil, cardamom, and frankincense and lavender oil.

Citronella Oil

Citronella oil comes from the grass of the *Cymbopogon nardus* plant. It has a grassy, earthy fragrance with hints of sweet citrus. If you've ever used a citronella candle to keep bugs away, you know what citronella oil smells like. It's usually devoid of color, but may have a slight yellow or amber tint to it. This strong oil contains geraniol and citronellal and can be a strong dermal irritant to those with sensitive skin. It's rarely applied topically and has to be diluted heavily when it is. Avoid use of citronella oil when pregnant or if you have sensitive skin.

The main use for citronella essential oil is as an insect repellent. It can be added to a spray bottle and sprayed on surfaces you want to keep free of insects or it can be diffused into a room to clear the room of bugs. It can also be added to candles that can be burnt outdoors to keep flies, bees and mosquitoes away. When used outdoors, multiple candles will be needed. It's best to surround the area you want to keep free of bugs. Dab it onto a cotton ball and apply it to the neck area of pets to keep fleas and ticks from latching on.

While the main use for citronella oil is to keep insects away, there are other uses for the oil. It has the following properties associated with it:

- **Antibacterial.**
- **Antiseptic.**
- **Deodorant.**
- **Insecticide.**
- **Parasitic.**
- **Stimulant.**

- **Tonic.**

Diffuse citronella oil into a room to provide mental clarity and focus. It can also be used to get rid of foul odors and may help ease symptoms of the common cold. To be honest with you, these attributes can be better-achieved with other oils and the main use of citronella oil is to keep bugs away.

Citronella oil is more often than not used on its own, but can be blended with other oils. Citrus oils, cedarwood and lavender oil work well when blended with citronella.

Coriander Oil

Coriander essential oil is typically referred to as coriander seed oil because it's distilled from the seeds of the coriander plant. It has a spicy, woody scent not unlike that of the spice used for cooking, which is made from the same seeds. The oil is clear to light yellow in color and is of thin viscosity. It's used quite a bit in aromatherapy and has seen use in perfumes, toiletries and homemade soaps.

The following properties have been attributed to coriander oil:

- **Analgesic.**
- **Antibacterial.**
- **Antifungal.**
- **Antirheumatic.**
- **Antispasmodic.**
- **Aphrodisiac.**
- **Carminative.**
- **Depurative.**
- **Digestive.**
- **Stimulant.**
- **Stomachic.**
- **Tonic.**

Coriander oil can be diffused or it can be added to a carrier oil blend and massaged into the skin. There are no known contraindications and it's generally regarded as safe. As is the case with all essential oils, it could be a dermal irritant to those with sensitive skin, so always test it in a small area before broader application.

The main applications of coriander seed oil are for stress relief and to alleviate mental fatigue. This effect is only seen when smaller amounts of the oil are used, as larger amounts have been known to make people groggy and less aware of their surroundings. Coriander seed oil can be diluted and applied topically to provide some relief from aches and pains and may stop muscle spasms in their tracks. Topical application can also be used to cut down on the odors normally associated with sweating.

The aphrodisiac qualities of this oil can stimulate the hormones that increase attraction and get you in the right mood. Those who use coriander oil for this purpose typically use it as a marital aid to increase libido and revamp interest in sex.

The fragrance of coriander seed oil lends itself well to blending and it works well with a number of other oils. Citrus oils, cardamom seed, cinnamon, frankincense, nutmeg, pine, ylang ylang and most wood oils all can be blended with coriander oil to good effect.

Eucalyptus Oil

There are more than a thousand different types of eucalyptus trees found across the globe, a handful of which eucalyptus oil can be obtained from. *Eucalyptus globulus* is the most common and is the type of oil referred to in this chapter when "eucalyptus oil" is mentioned. The oil is distilled from the leaves and twigs of the tree and features a fresh, campherous fragrance that has a bit of a bite to it. It's clear to light yellow in color and is of thin consistency.

Eucalyptus oil features the following properties:

- **Analgesic.**
- **Antibacterial.**
- **Antifungal.**
- **Antineuralgic.**
- **Antirheumatic.**
- **Antiseptic.**
- **Antispasmodic.**
- **Antiviral.**
- **Decongestant.**
- **Deodorant.**
- **Depurative.**
- **Diuretic.**
- **Expectorant.**
- **Febrifuge.**
- **Stimulant.**
- **Vulnerary.**

Eucalyptus oil is considered a cooling oil that can be used to help with minor fevers and is one of the oils commonly used to relieve aches and pains. The cooling effect also works well on sunburns, but it should only be used on minor sunburns where there's no blistering and the skin isn't broken. Respiratory issues can be eased by diffusing eucalyptus oil or diluting it with carrier oil and rubbing it onto the chest. It helps clear congestion and may even be able to help clear up a stuffy head due to allergies or the common cold. Some people claim to have used it to ease the effects of asthma, but only use it for this purpose under the watchful eye of your healthcare provider.

While it isn't quite as effective an insect repellent as citronella oil, eucalyptus oil will repel insects. For best results, combine it with citronella oil to hit pests with a one-two punch that'll send them running out the room it's diffused in. For insect bites that won't stop itching, try dabbing a tiny amount of neat eucalyptus oil directly onto the bite.

Combine 5 drops of eucalyptus and 10 drops of lavender oil with a quart of water to create healthy and natural dishwashing liquid that can be used to clean your dishes and leave them smelling fresh. It can also be added to liquid castile soap along with lemon essential oil and used as a general-purpose cleaner that can be used on hard surfaces around the house.

Avoid eucalyptus oil while pregnant or if you have high blood pressure or are epileptic. Be very careful and dilute this potent oil heavily before applying it to the skin. It's a strong oil and can be a dermal irritant. While it's rarely a good idea to take essential oils internally, eucalyptus oil is especially toxic and internal consumption should be avoided at all costs.

You can blend eucalyptus oil with a number of other oils, but you're definitely going to know it's in there. Wood oils and citrus oils blend well with eucalyptus oil.

Lemon Eucalyptus Oil

Lemon eucalyptus is another essential oil that comes from the eucalyptus tree, this time from the *Eucalyptus citriodora* tree. The oil is distilled from the leaves and the twigs of the tree and instead of smelling campherous like regular eucalyptus oil, it has a deep, lemony fragrance. This is due to the fact that lemon eucalyptus oil contains less eucalyptol, the compound that gives eucalyptus its signature fragrance, than regular eucalyptus oil. Lemon eucalyptus oil ranges from clear to pale yellow in color.

The following properties are associated with lemon eucalyptus oil:

- **Antibacterial.**
- **Antifungal.**
- **Antiseptic.**
- **Antiviral.**
- **Calming.**
- **Deodorant.**
- **Expectorant.**
- **Insecticidal.**

Lemon eucalyptus oil can be diffused into a room to help ease the effects of respiratory infection. Those with colds and flus that feature a cough as one of the symptoms may benefit from the expectorant properties of lemon eucalyptus. Heavily dilute the oil with carrier oil and rub it onto your chest for more relief. It can also be rubbed into sore or spasming muscles. Some research has shown it to be effective against toenail fungus. Apply it to the affected area until the fungus clears up.

When diluted and applied directly to the skin, lemon eucalyptus will deter mosquitoes and may keep ticks at bay as well. It's used as an alternative to DEET, but will need to be applied more frequently.

Use small amounts of lemon eucalyptus and always test it in a smaller area before applying it to a larger area. It can cause skin irritation and should not be taken internally because it's highly toxic when consumed. Pregnant women should not use lemon eucalyptus.

Regular eucalyptus oil has strong medicinal properties that aren't as defined when it comes to lemon eucalyptus. For this reason, many people opt to use eucalyptus over lemon eucalyptus unless they're using the lemon variety for its scent. Lemon eucalyptus is easier to blend with other oils because it isn't as overpoweringly-campherous, and it blends well with basil, clary sage, frankincense, lavender, tea tree and wood and citrus oils.

Frankincense

Most people have heard of frankincense because it's one of the Biblical oils that was brought to Baby Jesus as a gift from the wise menupon his birth. It ranks amongst the most popular oils used for aromatherapy purposes and is one of the oils all aromatherapy practitioners should have on hand. The oil is extracted from the resin of a tree known as the *Boswellia carteri* tree that grows in Somalia, Saudi Arabia and China. It has a hauntingly-rich balsamic scent that dances around your nose and lingers with you long after you move the bottle away. It can be either pale yellow or pale green in color and has a thin viscosity.

Frankincense is considered one of the more spiritual essential oils and is frequently diffused into rooms as a means of relaxing and getting in touch with one's inner self. It somehow manages to be energizing and uplifting while keeping you calm and grounded at the same time. Those who practice meditation can diffuse frankincense into the room during a meditation session to deepen their breathing and to help them get in the zone.

The benefits of frankincense oil aren't just spiritual. Frankincense oil has the following properties:

- Analgesic.
- **Antifungal.**
- **Anti-inflammatory.**
- **Antioxidant.**
- **Antiseptic.**
- **Astringent.**
- **Carminative.**

- **Digestive.**
- **Diuretic.**
- **Expectorant.**
- **Sedative.**
- **Tonic.**
- **Vulnerary.**

Frankincense is said to be an anti-aging oil that can help promote healing in aged or damaged skin. It can be diluted with carrier oil and rubbed into scars and stretch marks to help them fade away and is another oil that can be diffused into a room or rubbed into the chest to ease congestion and help open the airways of those suffering from respiratory conditions. A drop or two of frankincense oil can be added to oral care products and blended in to help prevent bad breath, tooth aches and possibly even cavities. Combine it with baking soda to create an all-natural toothpaste or with water to create a mouthwash that smells great and has antiseptic and antibacterial properties.

As you can see, frankincense is a very versatile oil, and it's one that's generally thought to be safe for use for most people. It does have emmenagogue properties, so avoid use of frankincense when pregnant or attempting to become pregnant.

The woody, balsamic fragrance of frankincense oil blends well with most essential oils. Try blending it with orange, lemon or sandalwood oil to see which you prefer.

Geranium Oil

Geranium essential oil comes from the flowers, leaves and stems of the geranium plant, one variety of which goes by the scientific name *Pelargonium odorantissimum*. There are roughly 10 varieties of geranium from which essential oil can be extracted. While you may be familiar with geraniums as a garden flower, the varieties of geraniums typically planted in gardens aren't good suppliers of essential oil. A higher-quality geranium oil can be obtained from the *Pelargonium roseum* plant and is referred to by most suppliers of essential oil as rose geranium oil because it smells like roses instead of the sweet, earthy floral scent normally associated with geranium oil.

Pure geranium oil is quite expensive, so some manufacturers dilute it with other similar, but less expensive, oils. That's not a huge problem when the oil is clearly labeled as an oil blend or as an adulterated oil, but there are some shady dealers out there who adulterate it and sell it as pure geranium oil. Keep this in mind when you come across a deal on geranium oil that seems too good to be true.

While geranium oil is highly-sought after for perfumes and high-end toiletries, it also features a number of beneficial properties, including the following:

- **Analgesic.**
- **Antibacterial.**
- **Antidepressant.**
- **Anti-inflammatory.**
- **Antiseptic.**
- **Astringent.**

- **Cicatrisant.**
- **Deodorant.**
- **Diuretic.**
- **Emmenagogue.**
- **Hepatic.**
- **Insecticide.**
- **Rubifacient.**
- **Sedative.**
- **Tonic.**
- **Vermifuge.**
- **Vulnerary.**

Diffused geranium oil has a balancing effect on the mind, body and soul. It helps smooth out jagged emotions and stimulates both the brain and the immune system. Minor stress and melancholy feelings often go away after use of geranium oil. Diffuse it in the evening before bed and wake up feeling energetic and refreshed.

When combined with carrier oil and rubbed into the skin, geranium oil balances sebum production and can help reduce the effects of aging. It's also shown some promise when used to heal wounds and regenerate skin damaged by acne or other skin conditions. Apply it to wounds or cuts to promote faster healing and to get minor cuts to clot up and stop bleeding. Geranium oil is astringent and its skin-tightening properties can be used to tighten up loose skin and temporarily eliminate or reduce wrinkles. It can also be used as a natural deodorant that goes straight to the source and eliminates the bacteria that cause body odor, both inside and outside the body.

Detoxify with geranium oil by applying it to your skin or diffusing it into a room you're sitting in. It's a diuretic and will help your body eliminate toxins via urination. Chemicals, sugars, heavy metals and a number of other toxins can all be eliminated during urination and it can help normalize the amount of sodium stored in the body.

Geranium oil also has mild insect-repellent properties, so rubbing diluted oil onto exposed areas before heading outside may keep mosquitoes and other insects at bay. Some people add several drops of geranium oil to shampoo and use it to get rid of head lice.

There's little worry of skin irritation when geranium oil is properly-diluted before application, but a small percentage of the population does experience irritation due to this oil. Avoid use of geranium oil while pregnant because it carries emmenagogue properties and theoretically could cause miscarriage.

Geranium oil is a commonly-used, albeit rather expensive, perfume oil that acts as a middle note in perfume blends. It blends well with most essential oils and is commonly combined with citrus oils, chamomile, clary sage, jasmine, patchouli, peppermint, sandalwood and ylang ylang.

Grapefruit Oil

As a child, I always disliked grapefruit because they were big and bitter and didn't smell or taste as good as the rest of the citrus fruits I enjoyed. I always cringed a little when my grandmother would ask me if I wanted a bite of grapefruit in the morning. My personal distaste for grapefruit as a food item kept me from trying grapefruit oil even though I'd heard of its many benefits. When I finally tried it, I was surprised to find it to be a pleasant addition to my daily routine.

Grapefruit essential oil is cold-pressed from the rinds of grapefruit and has a light, refreshing citrus scent that's used as a top note in a number of high-end perfumes. It has a viscosity similar to that of water and is yellow to light green in color. Some companies sell both white and pink grapefruit oil. The main difference is in the smell of the oil, as white grapefruit oil has a lighter fragrance that dissipates quickly, while pink grapefruit has a muskier, sweeter aroma that sticks around a little longer.

The following properties are associated with grapefruit oil:

- **Antibacterial.**
- **Antidepressant.**
- **Antiseptic.**
- **Astringent.**
- **Depurative.**
- **Digestive.**
- **Diuretic.**
- **Stimulant.**

- **Restorative.**

Try adding a few drops of grapefruit oil to your morning shower or bath to get you ready for the day. It helps to relieve stress and will leave you feeling happy and refreshed and is especially good for those days where you wake up feeling anxious or nervous about events that are taking place later on in the day. Diffusion is thought to assist with the removal of cellulite, but it may be more effective to dilute it and apply it topically to the area that needs work.

Combine 10 drops of grapefruit oil with a container of liquid castile soap to create an all-natural dishwashing soap. I like to add a few drops of lemon oil and a few drops of lavender oil as well. This same soap can be used to clean and disinfect hard surfaces throughout the house.

The phototoxicity of grapefruit oil is of concern when the oil is applied to an area of the body that's going to get direct sunlight. Avoid exposing skin that has had grapefruit oil applied to it to direct sunlight for 24 hours after application. Grapefruit oil can be a dermal irritant, so dilute it heavily before applying it topically and always test it in a small area.

Like most citrus oils, grapefruit oil lends itself well to blending and can be blended with a number of oils, including other citrus oils, black pepper, cardamom, clove, eucalyptus, frankincense, lavender, patchouli, peppermint and floral oils.

Jasmine Oil

Traditionally, the flowers of the jasmine plant were steam-distilled to produce very small amounts of jasmine essential oil that were put to use for aromatherapy purposes. Each jasmine plant only produces a few flowers and they each produce a miniscule amount of essential oil when distilled using traditional methods. Manufacturers today produce the oil through use of solvents, so true jasmine essential oil is all but impossible to find. Products labeled as "jasmine absolute" indicate a solvent was used to remove the oil from the flowers.

There are two types of jasmine from which essential oil can be obtained. *Jasminum grandiflora*, also known as Royal Jasmine, and *Jasminum officinale*, also known as Common Jasmine, both produce oils that can be labeled as jasmine essential oil. While there may be minor differences in the chemical composition between the two, they're pretty much the same when it comes to putting them to use for aromatherapy.

Jasmine essential oil has the following attributes:

- **Antibacterial.**
- **Antidepressant.**
- **Antiseptic.**
- **Antispasmodic.**
- **Aphrodisiac.**
- **Cicatrisant.**
- **Emmenagogue.**
- **Expectorant.**
- **Galactagogue.**

- **Sedative.**

Inhaling the fragrance of jasmine oil is calming and uplifting and may help ward off depression. It uplifts the spirits and puts those who inhale it in a better mood, making them feel better about themselves and others. When you have a cold or respiratory tract infection, jasmine oil can be inhaled to provide relief from congestion and to help clear up a cough. Combine that with the ability of the oil to aid with sleep and you've got a potent cold remedy that will help you sleep through the night.

Jasmine oil is also said to have aphrodisiac qualities, but it's unclear whether this is fact or a misconception. For best results, try combining jasmine with other known aphrodisiac oils like sandalwood and patchouli.

Dilute jasmine oil and apply it to wounds to take advantage of the antibacterial and antiseptic properties. It helps fight off infections and prevents wounds from turning septic. Once a wound has healed, jasmine oil can be used help eliminate scarring and it has seen use as a remedy for acne scars and stretch marks.

While jasmine oil is said to help women through the birthing process, it has emmenagogue properties and shouldn't be used by pregnant women prior to going into labor. It can cause an allergic reaction in people who are sensitive to jasmine and skin sensitization can occur if too much of this oil is used. Oil that's been extracted through use of solvents shouldn't be applied topically because the solvents can soak into the skin along with the oil.

Jasmine oil blends well with citrus oils, wood oils and most floral oils. An expensive, but potent, blend can be made by combining jasmine and rose oil.

Lavender Oil

There's good reason lavender essential oil is the most popular essential oil in existence. It's an inexpensive and versatile oil that has a large number of applications. Lavender oil is one of the few oils that's mild enough to where it can be applied neat by most people. Oddly enough, while lavender oil is the most popular essential oil by far, most people don't care for the smell the first time they breathe it in. Don't be surprised if you don't fall in love with it right away. It usually takes a handful of encounters before you fall in love with the sweet, floral fragrance of lavender.

Lavender oil comes from the flowers of the lavender bush. *Lavandula augustifolia* is the plant lavender oil is most commonly extracted from, but essential oil can also be taken from *Lavandula officinalis* or *Lavandula vera*. The oils drawn from those plants will have a slightly-different smell, but the properties will be similar.

Don't confuse spike lavender oil with lavender oil. It's cheaply produced and doesn't have the same benefits as lavender oil. Lavandin oil is a blend of lavender oil and spike lavender oil and is harsher than lavender oil. It's preferred by soap and body product makers because the smell is stronger, but it should be avoided by those looking to reap the benefits of lavender oil. Some sources indicate that it can actually make burns and skin problems worse instead of helping heal them like lavender oil will.

Lavender essential oil has been found to have the following properties:

- **Analgesic.**

- **Anticonvulsant.**
- **Antidepressant.**
- **Antihistamine.**
- **Anti-inflammatory.**
- **Antimicrobial.**
- **Antiseptic.**
- **Antitumor.**
- **Antiviral.**
- **Calming.**
- **Deodorant.**
- **Pain relief.**
- **Relaxing.**
- **Soothing.**

There are a ton of applications for this oil. It's commonly used to ease aches and pains and can be applied to minor cuts and burns to help relieve pain and to promote healing. It also works well to relieve itching. If you have scars or stretch marks, lavender oil may be able to help lighten them and heal the damaged skin around them. When my kids get sunburnt, they practically beg for aloe vera and lavender oil because it quickly relieves the pain associated with all but the worst of sunburns. Do not apply lavender oil if blistering is present or if the skin is broken. Lavender oil is also effective on dry skin, chapped skin and skin that's damaged from eczema or dermatitis. Mix several drops of lavender oil with coconut oil and rub it into the affected area.

Lavender oil has deodorant properties. A few drops can be added to a spray bottle full of water to create a deodorant spray that can be used in a manner similar to Febreze.

One of my favorite tricks to get the family relaxed and ready for bed at night is to diffuse lavender into the family room while we're all winding down. This is especially effective on those nights where the family is particularly rambunctious and there's no end in sight to the energy level the kids are displaying. It works well to help soothe my frazzled nerves after a long day. I rub several drops of lavender oil between my palms and cup my hands over my mouth while inhaling slowly and deeply. I've been known to rub a drop or two of lavender oil into my pillow before I go to bed at night to help me sleep through the night. I can't say for sure it's the lavender oil, but the nights I rub it into the pillow, I wake up feeling refreshed and happy.

While there are definite safety concerns you need to be aware of with some of the stronger oils, lavender oil is a mild oil and rarely causes problems for those who use it. It's a great starter oil that will allow you reap the benefits of essential oils while learning how to harness their powers. There is still the slight risk of skin irritation, but lavender is one oil most people can handle.

Oddly enough, while lavender oil is one of the most beloved essential oils around, most people don't particularly like the smell the first time they try it. It grows on you and lavender oil will soon become one of your go-to oils when you realize its true power. As far as blending goes, lavender oil can be blended with almost any other oil. It really is that versatile.

Lemon Oil

Bend a lemon peel while looking closely at it and you'll see small geysers of liquid erupt from the pores in the peel. These geysers are lemon essential oil and they contain limonene, the chemical responsible for the fresh citrus aroma of lemons. Lemon essential oil is extracted from the peels via cold-pressing, which creates oil that ranges from light to deep yellow in color and has a thin viscosity.

The following properties have been associated with lemon oil:

- **Antibacterial.**
- **Antiseptic.**
- **Antiviral.**
- **Astringent.**
- **Disinfectant.**
- **Febrifuge.**
- **Haemostatic.**
- **Restorative.**

When it comes to using essential oils to scent household cleaning products, lemon oil is hard to beat. 10 to 20 drops of lemon oil added to a spray bottle full of water or liquid castile soap can be used as an all-purpose cleaner that cleans and disinfects most hard surfaces and will leave them smelling clean and fresh. Be aware that the lemon scent found in most commercial cleaners is a synthetic fragrance and doesn't carry with it the same benefits as lemon essential oil.

A drop of lemon oil applied to a bandage will keep wounds from getting infected, killing off bacterial and fungal growth. The strong antifungal capabilities of lemon oil make it a great choice for use to combat fungal infections like athletes foot and nail fungus. It can be diluted with carrier oil and massaged into sagging or weathered skin to rejuvenate it and tighten it up. Oily skin generally responds well to lemon oil because it slows excessive oil production and tightens up the pores. A mixture of water and a tiny amount of lemon oil can be used as mouthwash to help with mouth ulcers.

Diffuse lemon oil into rooms you want to deodorize and freshen. It won't just mask the odor like most commercial air fresheners. It actually eliminates the odor at the source. Diffused lemon essential calms you down and refreshes and reenergizes the mind while eliminating negative emotions. It also helps boost the immune system and cleanses the mind, the body and any surfaces it comes in contact with.

Lemon oil is known to be phototoxic, so avoid using it on areas of the body that are going to be exposed to the sun within 24 hours of application. The limonene in lemon essential oil may cause irritation or sensitization in people who have sensitive skin, so always dilute it and apply it with caution. Lemon essential oil doesn't keep well and will spoil quickly if it isn't stored in a dark container in a cool, dark place. Check the oil to make sure it isn't cloudy before you use it and don't apply cloudy lemon oil to your skin or you could suffer sensitization.

While lemon oil is commonly used on its own because of its fresh lemon scent, it can be blended with other citrus oils, wood oils and flower oils to create interesting and unique oil blends. I haven't found an oil yet that I didn't care for once I blended it with several drops of lemon oil, and that says a lot.

Lemon Balm (Melissa) Oil

Lemon balm oil is sold by some manufacturers under the moniker melissa oil because it comes from the leaves and flowers of the *Melissa officinalis* plant. It takes more than three tons of melissa to produce a pound of oil, so expect to pay a premium for pure melissa oil. A small bottle will run you upwards of $100, if you're able to find it at all. This steam-distilled oil is yellow to pale green in color and features fresh, lemony-citrus fragrance notes that are light and refreshing.

This powerful oil has the following properties associated with it:

- **Antibacterial.**
- **Anti-inflammatory.**
- **Antiseptic.**
- **Antispasmodic.**
- **Antiviral.**
- **Carminative.**
- **Diaphoretic.**
- **Digestive.**
- **Emmenagogue.**
- **Febrifuge.**
- **Nervine.**
- **Sedative.**
- **Sudorific.**
- **Tonic.**
- **Uterine.**
- **Vermifuge.**

Add 5 to 7 drops of lemon balm oil to a hot bath and soak in it while inhaling deeply to calm frayed nerves and soothe your soul. It brings peace and tranquility to the mind and may even slow your heartbeat a bit, helping carry you into a relaxed state. When panic starts to set in, several whiffs of lemon balm oil may be all that's needed to bring you back down to a normal level. Diffused lemon balm oil has seen use for relief from headaches and migraines.

Blend it with carrier oil and massage it into the skin to aid with fevers and upset stomachs. It can also be used to fight fungal infections and athlete's foot. This nervine oil serves as a general tonic for the nervous system and may play a role in keeping it functioning properly.

While it's generally considered nontoxic in low amounts, lemon balm oil is a warming oil that can cause skin irritation, so it shouldn't be applied at full strength. Avoid using large amounts of lemon balm oil and only use it occasionally when the situation calls for it. This isn't an oil that should be used as part of a daily aromatherapy routine. Lemon balm oil does have emmenagogue properties, so it's best avoided by pregnant women.

Since lemon balm oil is so expensive, most people choose to use it as part of a blend of other oils. It blends well with German chamomile, Roman chamomile, floral oils, frankincense and ylang ylang. I've also heard of people blending it with lavender oil to double up on the calming and soothing effect, which is a great idea when you're trying to wind down at the end of the day, but might not be in your best interest in the mornings if you've got a long day ahead of you.

Lemongrass Oil

Rounding out the lemon-scented oils is lemongrass, an oil that's steam-distilled from the grass of the *Cymbopogon flexuosus* or *Cymbopogon citratus* plants. The dark yellow oil features a light yet penetrating lemon fragrance that's stronger than that of lemon balm or lemon oil.

Lemongrass oil has the following properties:

- **Analgesic.**
- **Antibacterial.**
- **Antifungal.**
- **Antifungal.**
- **Anti-inflammatory.**
- **Antimicrobial.**
- **Antioxidant.**
- **Antiparasitic.**
- **Antiseptic.**
- **Antiviral.**
- **Astringent.**
- **Carminative.**
- **Deodorant.**
- **Digestive.**
- **Febrifuge.**
- **Insect repellent.**
- **Sedative.**
- **Tonic.**

Use lemongrass oil to wake up and reinvigorate yourself on those days where you're feeling tired, stressed or worn down. It works well for jet lag after a long flight and will revitalize the mind while helping the body along as well. Lemongrass oil can be heavily diluted with carrier oil and rubbed into cellulite to help attack it at the source. It can also be used as a general tonic that relieves everything from digestive issues to general aches and pains and is a great addition to natural skin and body care products like deodorants, acne creams, skin lotions and body wash. A few drops added to a natural shampoo blend will leave your hair looking shiny and lustrous. Take advantage of the antifungal properties of lemongrass oil by combining 5 drops of the oil with a few ounces of coconut or almond oil. Rub the oil into areas of your body like your feet and nails to get rid of fungus.

Diffuse lemongrass oil into a room to deodorize and clean the air in the room. You can get the same effect by adding 10 to 15 drops of oil to a spray bottle full of water, shaking it up and misting the room.

Combine lemongrass oil with other insect repellent oils like citronella to create oil blends that will work great to keep insects at bay. The oil blends can be diffused into rooms you want to keep free of bugs or you can dilute them with carrier oil and massage them into the skin to keep the bugs from biting while you're out and about.

Avoid lemongrass if you've got glaucoma. Be careful when applying it to the skin because it can cause sensitization and should never be applied to broken skin or an open wound. If you can find oil that's naturally low in citral, it'll lessen, but not completely eliminate the chance of a skin reaction at the expense of some of the effectiveness of the oil.

There are a lot of essential oils lemongrass oil can be blended with. Other citrus oils work well, as do most floral, wood and spice oils. Lemongrass oil is one of the most versatile oils around when it comes to creating oil blends that are functional and smell great.

Lime Oil

Lime oil is either cold-pressed or steam-distilled from the peels of limes and has a sharp, slightly-sweet fragrance that's light and refreshing. If you've ever bent a lime peel back and forth and smelled the fresh scent of lime, that's exactly what you get from lime oil. This oil is readily available and it's one of the least-expensive essential oils in existence, so there's really no reason not to add it to your collection.

Don't let the fact that it doesn't break the bank turn you off. The price of an essential oil is usually tied to how hard it is to obtain the oil, not how beneficial it is. Lime oil has a number of therapeutic qualities, including the following:

- **Antibacterial.**
- **Antibacterial.**
- **Antiseptic.**
- **Antispasmodic.**
- **Antiviral.**
- **Astringent.**
- **Carminative.**
- **Deodorant.**
- **Febrifuge.**

Add lime oil to a diffuser along with your other favorite citrus oils and the lime oil in the blend will leave you feeling energized and fresh. It cheers up dark and gloomy moods while purifying both the air in the room and your cloudy spirit.

Dilute lime oil with carrier oil and massage it into the skin to cool down fevers from colds or the flu. It can also be used to help ease pain associated with arthritis or sore muscles and its astringent action makes it a good choice for people who have acne due to oily skin. Add several drops of lime oil to a warm bath and soak in it while inhaling the steam to help with respiratory issues. External application of lime oil can help prevent infections and will protect wounds against sepsis.

The phototoxicity of lime oil is of concern when it's applied to areas of the body that will be exposed to sunlight. Wait at least 24 hours before exposing the area where the oil was applied to the sun. Lime oil can be a dermal irritant, so use caution when applying it to the skin. Some sources state that lime oil that's steam-distilled doesn't have the same phototoxicity or risk of irritation as oil that's been cold-pressed.

Blend lime oil with other citrus oils, lavender or ylang ylang oil to create oil blends that smell great and combine the effects of the oils.

Myrrh

Myrrh and frankincense have been in use for tens of thousands of years and myrrh is one of the Biblical oils given to Jesus by the three wise men in the Bible. Myrrh essential oil is distilled from the resin of the *Commiphora myrrha* bush. The golden brown oil has an earthy, balsamic fragrance that punches right into your nasal cavity on its own, but works well when blended with other wood oils, citrus oils, lavender or chamomile.

The following properties have been associated with myrrh oil:

- **Antifungal.**
- **Anti-inflammatory.**
- **Antimicrobial.**
- **Antiseptic.**
- **Astringent.**
- **Balsamic.**
- **Carminative.**
- **Cicatrisant.**
- **Digestive.**
- **Emmenagogue.**
- **Expectorant.**
- **Sedative.**
- **Stimulant.**
- **Stomachic.**
- **Tonic.**
- **Vulnerary.**

Diffuse myrrh oil or dilute it and rub it on your chest to help clear up congestion associated with colds and respiratory tract infections. Add myrrh oil to a cold compress and use it on minor wounds, scrapes and burns. Once the wounds have healed, continue applying myrrh oil to help eliminate scarring. Use the antifungal properties of myrrh to your advantage by applying it to areas where fungal infections are occurring. It works well to combat athlete's foot and nail fungus, just to name a couple.

If you're having trouble sleeping at night, diffuse myrrh oil into your room or add a couple drops of oil to the back side of your pillow. Myrrh has a sedative effect and breathing the aroma of myrrh may be all you need to help you drift off and stay asleep through the night.

Combine a couple drops of myrrh oil with a drop of cardamom seed oil to create a natural mouthwash that will help eliminate ulcers and will leave your breath smelling fresh for hours. Be careful not to swallow the mouthwash, as myrrh oil can be toxic when large enough amounts are ingested. Pregnant women should avoid myrrh oil altogether because of its emmenagogue properties.

Orange Blossom (Neroli) Oil

Neroli oil, also known as orange blossom oil, is steam-distilled from the blossoms of the orange tree and, along with lavender and tea tree oil, is one of the most popular essential oils in use for aromatherapy. The oil is dark brown in color and is of a medium-thick viscosity. It has a strong floral fragrance with hints of citrus and is one of the more exotic oils around. On its own, the fragrance can be overpowering and is almost sickly-sweet. This powerful oil is at its best when used in small amounts and blended with other floral or citrus oils.

It takes almost 100 pounds of orange blossoms to produce just a pound of neroli oil. Since it's expensive to make, it's often adulterated by manufacturers looking to maximize profit. Look for pure, unadulterated neroli oil for aromatherapy purposes.

The following benefits are attributed to neroli oil:

- **Antibacterial.**
- **Antifungal.**
- **Anti-inflammatory.**
- **Antiseptic.**
- **Antispasmodic.**
- **Aphrodisiac.**
- **Carminative.**
- **Cicatrisant.**
- **Cordial.**
- **Deodorant.**
- **Sedative.**
- **Tonic.**

Diffused neroli oil has a relaxing, almost sedative, effect that mellows out the body and mind. It isn't a great oil to use when you need to be sharp and focused, so it's best used in the evenings or during a meditation session. Sufferers of insomnia often use neroli oil to help them drift off to sleep. The diffused oil can be used to relieve headaches and to ease nervous tension. A couple drops combined with a tablespoon of almond oil can be rubbed into the base of the neck to get rid of migraines. Combine neroli and lavender in a spray bottle full of water to create a deodorant spray that will eliminate even the strongest of odors. I spray this mixture into my son's gym bag and it always smells fresh and clean, even after he gets home from football practice.

Add the oil to a bath and soak in it to unwind after a long day. It'll help your skin regenerate and rebuild. Massage the oil into scars and stretch marks to help them fade away.

Unlike citrus oils derived from the peels of citrus fruit, neroli oil isn't considered a phototoxic oil and no special precautions need to be taken to avoid sunlight after application.

Patchouli Oil

When it comes to exotic essential oils, patchouli oil takes the cake. It comes from a tropical plant known to the scientific world as *Pogostemon cablin*, or *Pogostemon patchouli*. The oil is steam-distilled from the leaves of the plant and is a thick, dark brown oil that feels oily to the touch and leaves behind a greasy residue. Patchouli oil is harsh when fresh, but it gets better as it ages like a fine wine, and it mellows out and becomes sweeter and easier on the nose. If you open a bottle of patchouli oil and don't like its smell, don't throw it out. Seal it tight, give it time to age and check it again later on down the road. You might be surprised to find the oil smells much better than you remember.

Patchouli oil is a strange oil in that most people don't like it the first time they take in its rich, fragrant aroma. Once they get used to it, patchouli oil usually becomes a go-to oil thanks to its many benefits, including the following:

- **Antidepressant.**
- **Antifungal.**
- **Antiseptic.**
- **Aphrodisiac.**
- **Astringent.**
- **Cicatrisant.**
- **Deodorant.**
- **Diuretic.**
- **Febrifuge.**
- **Insect repellent.**

- **Sedative.**
- **Tonic.**

Patchouli oil is a great oil to diffuse or to add to a hot bath to help you wind down after a long day. It levels out your emotions and creates feelings of happiness and contentment. It's thought of as a peaceful oil, which shouldn't come as a surprise since patchouli was a favorite amongst hippies and activists in the 60's and 70's.

The antifungal and antibacterial properties of this oil are strong, so it can be used to fight infection and to promote the healing of minor cuts, scrapes and burns. It also promotes the growth of new skin cells and is a good choice for eliminating stubborn scars and stretch marks. Dilute patchouli oil with carrier oil and massage it into dry, cracked skin or skin that's been damaged by acne or eczema to help it clear up. Patchouli oil doesn't just repel insects, which it does surprisingly well; it's also a great oil to dab on insect bites to stop them from itching or burning.

Patchouli oil is considered safe for most people to use. It can be used on its own or combined with other oils like citrus oils, wood oils, cinnamon, clary sage, frankincense, and lavender, myrrh or rose oil.

Peppermint Oil

Peppermint oil is one oil most people should be familiar with. It smells like peppermint candy, albeit much more intense. The oil is typically steam-distilled from the flowers and leaves of the plant and is a clear yellow color.

While peppermint oil isn't to be taken lightly, it does have a number of benefits, including the following:

- **Analgesic.**
- **Antibacterial.**
- **Antifungal.**
- **Anti-inflammatory.**
- **Antimicrobial.**
- **Antiseptic.**
- **Antispasmodic.**
- **Astringent.**
- **Carminative.**
- **Cholagogue.**
- **Digestive.**
- **Emmenagogue.**
- **Expectorant.**
- **Febrifuge.**
- **Insect repellent.**
- **Nervine.**
- **Stimulant.**
- **Stomachic.**
- **Vermifuge.**

The menthol content of the oil is responsible for a large number of the benefits and is the reason why the oil produces an immediate cooling sensation when inhaled. When applied topically, it promotes blood flow to the area of application, opening up the tiny capillaries in the area. If you've ever applied Vick's Vapor rub to sore muscles, application of peppermint oil has the same effect. The cooling effect of the menthol in the oil provides pain relief and can reduce swelling and inflammation. It has strong antifungal properties and can be used to eliminate nail fungus and athlete's foot.

Diffuse peppermint oil into a room or inhale steam containing peppermint oil to clear up congestion and to relieve headaches. It provides instant relief from respiratory issues, but the relief is usually short-lived. Peppermint oil is a stimulant, so it can provide clarity of mind and may eliminate feelings of nausea. It can also be used for stress relief and to relieve the effects of mental exhaustion and jet lag.

A few drops of peppermint oil can be added to a glass of water to create natural mouthwash that cleans and disinfects. It helps eliminate harmful bacteria in the mouth and gums and can be added to natural toothpaste to leave your mouth clean and your breath smelling minty fresh.

While the smell of peppermint oil is familiar, be aware this is a powerful oil that can irritate the mucous membranes and is toxic to the nerves in larger amounts. Epileptics and pregnant women should avoid this oil. It can cause sensitization and skin irritation, so always dilute it heavily and test it on a small area prior to applying it to a larger area.

Peppermint oil blends well with floral oils, citrus oils and can be combined with citronella oil to keep insects away.

Rose Otto Oil

Pure rose otto oil commands a premium price because it takes more than 50,000 roses to create a single ounce of steam-distilled rose oil. Rose absolute is slightly less-expensive because solvent is used to extract the oil and the yield is greater. Rose otto oil is preferable to rose absolute for aromatherapy purposes because trace amounts of the solvent is left behind in rose absolute.

Rose otto oil has the following therapeutic properties:

- **Antibacterial.**
- **Antidepressant.**
- **Antiseptic.**
- **Antispasmodic.**
- **Antiviral.**
- **Aphrodisiac.**
- **Astringent.**
- **Cicatrisant.**
- **Depurative.**
- **Emmenagogue.**
- **Hepatic.**
- **Laxative.**
- **Stomachic.**
- **Tonic.**

Common in expensive perfumes, rose oil smells exactly like what you'd expect concentrated roses to smell like. It has a soothing quality to it that harmonizes the emotions and balances one's mental state of mind. It eases harsh emotions like anger, fear and depression, and is a great oil to use when you're having trouble sorting through your emotions.

Rose oil moisturizes and stimulates the skin when applied topically and is considered a good oil for most skin types. It can be used to relieve inflammation, headaches, migraines and redness or irritation of the skin. Women can use it to help with menstrual or menopausal issues, but it should be avoided by pregnant women because of its emmenagogue qualities.

There are a number of oils rose oil can be combined with to create great-smelling oil blends, but it's really an oil that works well on its own. If you can afford rose oil, it's a great oil to have on hand.

Tea Tree Oil

If your budget only allows for a few oils to be kept on-hand, tea tree oil is one of the oils you're going to want. It's derived from the leaves of the tea tree, which goes by scientific name *Melaleuca alternifolia* and is native to Australia. The medicinal, herbaceous fragrance of this thin, yellow oil is going to take some getting used to, but most people learn to love it once they start to realize the many benefits of tea tree oil.

Tea tree oil has the following properties associated with it:

- **Analgesic.**
- **Antibacterial.**
- **Antifungal.**
- **Anti-inflammatory.**
- **Antimicrobial.**
- **Antiparasitic.**
- **Antiseptic.**
- **Antiviral.**
- **Decongestant.**
- **Deodorant.**
- **Diaphoretic.**
- **Expectorant.**
- **Insect repellent.**
- **Stimulant.**
- **Vulnerary.**

We have a running joke around my house when anyone complains of an illness or ailment. My husband and I look at each other and both say, "Just rub some tea tree oil on it." While we do this to be funny, there is some truth to it because tea tree oil is a versatile oil with a wide variety of healing properties. It can be used for bacterial and fungal issues, viruses, colds and flus. It helps the body fight off infections, knocks down inflammation and is great for congestion, coughs and fevers.

Add a few drops of tea tree oil to a tablespoon of carrier oil and rub it into abscesses, rashes, diaper rash, cold sores and sunburns to provide relief and promote healing. It can be used on mild burns and wounds and can help remove scarring and blemishes that are left behind. Tea tree oil can even be added to shampoo to help prevent dandruff and to moisturize dry scalp.

Several drops of tea tree oil in a glass of water can be used as mouthwash for ulcers, tonsillitis, throat and gum infections. Tea tree oil kills the bacteria that cause bad breath and will leave your breath smelling fresh and herbaceous.

While topical application and diffusion is considered safe, avoid consumption of tea tree oil. Tea tree oil is non-toxic and safe for most people to use, but can cause skin irritation in some people. It blends well with most essential oils. Floral oils like lavender, geranium and rose are some of my personal favorites.

The End

This is the end of the book, but hopefully it isn't the end of your journey into the world of essential oils. They truly are powerful essences and I believe they have the ability to change lives. The oils outlined here are some of the most popular oils, but they're really just the tip of the iceberg when it comes to the many plant oils there are available today.

I sincerely hope you enjoyed reading this book as much as I've enjoyed writing it. Until next time, folks.

Made in the USA
Lexington, KY
28 November 2016